IMAGINE YOU
ARE AN
ALUMINUM
ATOM

IMAGINE YOU ARE AN

ALUMINUM ATOM

DISCUSSIONS

WITH

MR. ALUMINUM

CHRISTOPHER EXLEY, PhD, FRSB

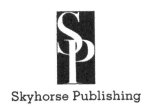

Skyhorse Publishing

Copyright © 2020 by Christopher Exley, PhD, FRSB

All rights reserved. No part of this book may be reproduced in any manner without the express written consent of the publisher, except in the case of brief excerpts in critical reviews or articles. All inquiries should be addressed to Skyhorse Publishing, 307 West 36th Street, 11th Floor, New York, NY 10018.

Skyhorse Publishing books may be purchased in bulk at special discounts for sales promotion, corporate gifts, fund-raising, or educational purposes. Special editions can also be created to specifications. For details, contact the Special Sales Department, Skyhorse Publishing, 307 West 36th Street, 11th Floor, New York, NY 10018 or info@skyhorsepublishing.com.

Skyhorse® and Skyhorse Publishing® are registered trademarks of Skyhorse Publishing, Inc.®, a Delaware corporation.

Visit our website at www.skyhorsepublishing.com.

10 9 8 7 6 5 4 3 2

Library of Congress Cataloging-in-Publication Data is available on file.

Cover design by Daniel Brount

Print ISBN: 978-1-5107-6253-4
Ebook ISBN: 978-1-5107-6254-1

Printed in the United States of America

TABLE OF CONTENTS

Chapter 1: Why Have I Written a Book on Aluminum?   1

Chapter 2: Why Am I Worried about Aluminum?   5

Chapter 3: Some Simple Aluminum Biochemistry   10

Chapter 4: Where Is Aluminum in the Body?   14

Chapter 5: Measuring the Body Burden of Aluminum   18

    Let's Start with Hair   19

    What About Blood?   20

    We Advocate Urine   21

    Urine Sampling to Estimate the Body Burden of Aluminum   23

Chapter 6: Aluminum In Doesn't Equal Aluminum Out   25

Chapter 7: I Am the Aluminum I Eat (or Am I?)   30

Chapter 8: Live Safely and Effectively in the Aluminum Age   33

    Food and Drink   33

    Medication   37

    Cosmetics and Personal Care Products   39

    Social Habits   41

    The Air We Breathe   44

    Getting Aluminum Out of the Body   45

Chapter 9: A Silicon-Rich Mineral Water a Day Keeps . . .
Aluminum at Bay   48

    Early Days   48

    Back to Today   49

Chapter 10: Pregnancy and Why Infant Exposure to Aluminum
Is a Special Case   61

Chapter 11: Tell Me Again Why There Is Aluminum in Vaccines   72

Chapter 12: Aluminum Is a Cause of and Contributor to
Human Disease   89

Chapter 13: What We Need to Know about Aluminum
in Human Brain Tissue   93

Chapter 14: Alzheimer's Disease and the Aluminum Elephant
in the Room   95

Chapter 15: Building a Case for Aluminum and Breast Cancer   104

Chapter 16: Aluminum Is a Genuine Contender as a Cause of
Multiple Sclerosis   108

Chapter 17: A Top Trumps Mechanism of Aluminum Toxicity   112

Chapter 18: Camelford—Anatomy of a Government Cover-up   117

   Aluminum and Camelford   119

Chapter 19: Politics   127

   Letter to the Editor   132

   *Letter to the Editor of Academic Pediatrics: The Safety of Aluminum
   Adjuvants in Infants*   139

   Closer to Home   142

Chapter 20: Imagine You Are an Aluminum Atom   147

Acknowledgments   151

To Olya

IMAGINE YOU
ARE AN
ALUMINUM
ATOM

CHAPTER 1

Why Have I Written a Book on Aluminum?

While the idea of writing this book has been gestating in my mind for some time, I only started to put words on paper as the Earth caught a cold from COVID-19. As I write, I am reminded of the book title *Love in the Time of Cholera*; not, of course, in comparing myself to Gabriel García Márquez and certainly not in a comparison of diseases. However, as the current "pandemic" unfolds and its true identity is revealed, I am reminded that fear is the key to controlling the narrative. I do not wish to go down this road in this book. I am not looking to scare anyone. I am hoping to inform as many as may wish to be informed about aluminum and its impact upon our lives. That said and back to the aforementioned Gabriel García Márquez, I am writing a love story, of sorts, and I am in the midst of global chaos wrapped up and delivered by Bill Gates's World Health Organization (rarely was an organization more inappropriately named) and partners as a pandemic. At this moment in time, my university has closed all science buildings, and all my research is in limbo. The withdrawal symptoms I feel from not being able to continue with our work are far worse than any cold, even for an aging asthmatic like me. As an amputee is said to feel their missing limb, my missing research nags me continuously, and, realistically, this feeling is the backdrop to the words that I am endeavoring to write for you in this book. Writing about science can only ever be secondary to the joy of doing it. But I am going to give it a go!

I say that I am writing a love story because my pursuit of the understanding of aluminum's role in life and living has occupied all my working days. Without love, without passion, my aluminum crush would have passed long, long ago. Indeed, many whom I respect and admire have, on numerous occasions over the years, encouraged me to consider a quick divorce from aluminum. In doing so they were only thinking of my well-being and my academic career, though I am sure that they expected their advice to fall on deaf ears. Persistence, indeed pursuance, in science needs an appreciation, if not a love, of the subject and, for most, some acknowledgment of effort by your peers. The latter proves most elusive. While over thirty-five years of continuous effort have afforded me the luxury of the label of "Mr. Aluminum," in truth it often feels like I am the person who knows most about something that few are really interested in knowing about. In scientific circles, aluminum—in relation to human health specifically—has gone the way of the dinosaurs, though unlike dinosaurs there has not yet been a popular revival. Perhaps the resurgence is about to begin? Each waking day I continue my quest to understand aluminum in all living things, my Holy Grail, because I believe that it is the greatest untold story of science, and, yes, it is belief that continues to nurture my fascination and not a vain hope that my scientific peers will one day reward my efforts. Alas, the subject of my research alone dictates that there be no future trip to Stockholm or even The Royal Society of London to receive accolades for my efforts. However, please do believe me when I say that other forms of recognition from myriad individuals across the globe leave a smile on my face and a determination to continue and succeed in bringing scientific truth to light.

To date, I have written over 200 scientific papers, and it might be assumed that this should stand me in good stead for writing a book.[1] In reality, for me writing about aluminum has never been easy and straightforward, as almost every word is loaded with meaning. In writing a scientific paper, you are always cautious that your words accurately reflect the data, the results of the research, and that you leave, purposefully, any wider interpretation to the reader. A famous example of this, and I say famous as the paper in question has been downloaded from the journal website a staggering one million times, is our paper on aluminum in brain tissue in autism.[2] In writing this paper, we used the word vaccine only once, and

1 Publications of the Research Group, "Bioinorganic Chemistry of Aluminium & Silicon," https://www.keele.ac.uk/aluminium/publications/.

2 Matthew Mold, Dorcas Umar, Andrew King, and Christopher Exley, "Aluminium in brain tissue in autism," *Journal of Trace Elements in Medicine and Biology* 46 (March 2018): 7-82, https://www.sciencedirect.com/science/article/pii/S0946672X17308763?via%3Dihub.

this was in the paper's introduction in relation to other scientists' research. Nevertheless, this paper saw me christened by various Internet trolls, such as the notorious David Gorski, as being antivaccine. It heralded attacks on my person by the media, often inanely supported by press stooges masquerading as scientists. Google still offers "Christopher Exley Quack" as a viable search option. Nevertheless, it is an important, probably seminal, paper, and if you have not read it yet, then I recommend you join the million or so who have and download it from the journal website found in footnote 2.

Every word in every scientific paper I have written has always mattered to me because the subject matters to me. It is critically important to me that written information on aluminum be correct and supported by scientific data. I am not writing about beliefs or opinions; these are there, but only in what remains unwritten. I want you to read my words and from them distill my opinions, subtly disguised perhaps, as your own. Writing about aluminum is tough for me because I am afraid of passing on a wrong or ill-defined message. As you might imagine, this also makes me an obstinate reviewer of work by others on aluminum. In peer review, I reject many more manuscripts than I recommend for publication. I am sure that there are many willing to testify to my obstinacy and perhaps some who wreak their revenge when the opportunity is presented to them. I know that I reap what I sow, and I am comfortable with this. I am not reviewing the science of aluminum in this book. If you are a fellow scientist, even a member of the Aluminum Family, do not look for a direct citation of your work in this book. You are unlikely to find such, though you may still see your important research referenced in my thoughtful meanderings. I pride myself in having read almost every paper on aluminum published since about 1980 in mainstream academic journals. Those who have visited me at Keele University will recall an office bestrewn with box files replete with papers on aluminum. I have learned more about aluminum in living systems than I thought possible when I began my quest. I am expressing this learning herein. I am going to have a conversation with you about aluminum, and everything I tell you will be supported by published scientific literature.

I also want this book to be helpful. Every day without exception I receive emails asking me all manner of questions about aluminum. I hope that by writing this book I will give readers both knowledge and resources to investigate the answers to these questions. One of the possible subtitles I considered for the book, "Frequently Answered Questions," reflects this aim of the book. I will always make myself available to fill in the gaps, but I want everyone who is truly interested to read a little more deeply and to find for themselves not only answers, but also mystery, the latter being what continues to keep the subject of human exposure to aluminum alive and kicking.

CHAPTER 2

Why Am I Worried about Aluminum?

Why do we all need to know a little bit more about aluminum? Do we need a self-help guide for living in what I have coined "The Aluminum Age"?[1] What is it about aluminum that makes it different, even, I would say, special? What about iron, copper, or any of the so-called "heavy metals" like mercury, cadmium, or lead? Why must we pay particular attention to aluminum? Why, because its biogeochemistry—its natural history—raises two red flags immediately and simultaneously. Two danger signals that actually are easily missed by all of us and easily dismissed by those whose interests are conflicted by aluminum's omnipresence in human life and, consequently, are purposely blind to its danger signals. First, aluminum in all of its myriad forms is superabundant; it is the third most abundant element (after oxygen and silicon) of the Earth's crust. The land upon which we walk and the mountains we endeavor to climb are made of aluminum, silicon, and oxygen.[2] Second, aluminum is superreactive; it is both chemically and biologically reactive. However, these two red flags identify a paradox, as the abundant and biologically reactive aluminum has no biological function

---

1 Christopher Exley, "The Aluminium Age," *The Hippocratic Post*, March 21, 2017, https://www.hippocraticpost.com/mens-health/the-aluminium-age/.

2 Christopher Exley, "A biogeochemical cycle for aluminium?" *Journal of Inorganic Biochemistry* 97, no, 1 (September 2003): 1-7, https://www.sciencedirect.com/science/article/pii/S0162013403002745?via%3Dihub.

either in any organism today or in any extinct biota from the evolutionary past. We know the latter to be true since aluminum left no biochemical footprints in the sands of evolutionary time. This means in practical terms that when we encounter aluminum in our everyday lives, our bodies only see aluminum as an impostor, something foreign, and something for which we have not been preprepared through biochemical evolution.[3] This in turn means that all of our encounters with aluminum are adventitious, random, and chaotic. There is no aluminum homeostasis, no protection against it, and no controlled elimination. I have not always been so aware of aluminum's rules of engagement with life and living things, and so one might forgive others whose days, like mine, are not spent pondering the natural history of aluminum, for missing these red flags. However, science moves on slowly and inexorably and does now inform us of these facts about aluminum in as unequivocal a manner as science is able to work. After all, we do now accept that planet Earth moves around the sun and not the opposite, as was believed to be the case for many centuries. The science of aluminum continues to evolve, though I am not convinced that humans will live through enough generations to see aluminum emerge as an essential, as opposed to toxic, element of life. Do not forget that the essential elements of life today such as oxygen and calcium were major toxins before being successful in supporting life through the process of natural selection. Darwin was so right in so many ways that he could never have supposed. I was happy in 2009, as part of the celebrations of Darwin's life (two hundred years since his birth) and major work (one hundred and fifty years since publication of *On the Origin of Species*), to be asked by a major biochemistry journal to review the essentiality of aluminum through the lens of Darwinian natural selection.

The natural history of aluminum and life is for telling on another day and not now in this book. However, it is one of the great stories that helps to explain why Earth is unique among millions of planets in thousands of galaxies. Planet Earth is the original green economy and ultimate example of recycling, and throughout the several billion years of its existence, it never allowed the movement of biologically reactive aluminum from the

---

3 Christopher Exley, "Darwin, natural selection and the biological essentiality of aluminium and silicon," *Trends in Biochemical Sciences* 34, no. 12 (December 1, 2009): 589-593, https://www.cell.com/trends/biochemical-sciences/fulltext/S0968-0004(09)00167-4?_returnURL=https%3A%2F%2Flinkinghub.elsevier.com%2Fretrieve%2Fpii%2FS0968000409001674%3Fshowall%3Dtrue.

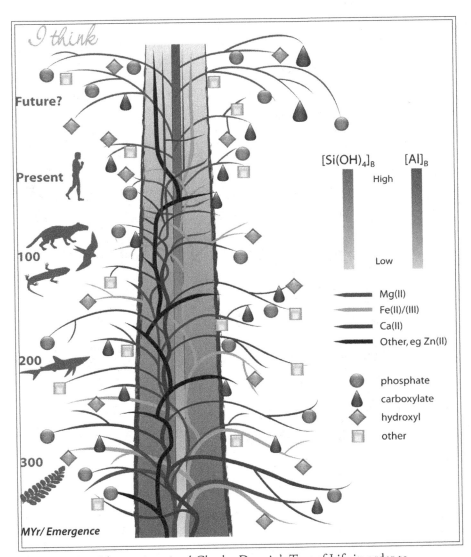

Figure 1. Here I have reimagined Charles Darwin's Tree of Life in order to demonstrate the emergence in evolutionary time of biologically reactive aluminum. Please see the full paper for a complete explanation.* (See color version in insert.)

* Ibid.

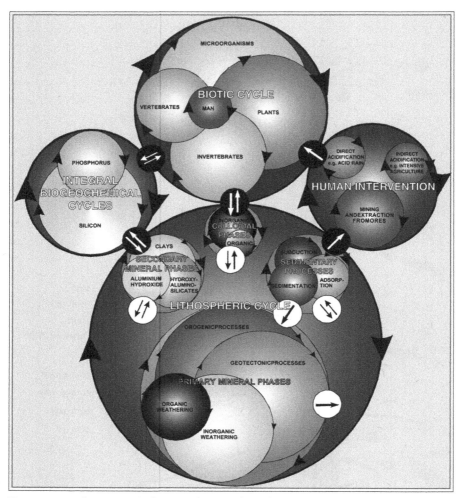

Figure 2. Aluminum's biogeochemical cycle ensured that almost no aluminum entered living things, the biotic cycle, until the advent of the Aluminum Age. Please see the full paper for a complete explanation of the cycle.** (See color version in insert.)

** Christopher Exley, "A biogeochemical cycle for aluminium?" Journal of Inorganic Biochemistry 97, no. 1 (September 15, 2003): 1-7, https://www.sciencedirect.com/science/article/pii/S0162013403002745?via%3Dihub.

geochemical cycle to the biotic—living—cycle. This glorious success in keeping aluminum out of all living things is summarized as a biogeochemical cycle recently circumvented by one significant caveat, the emergence of Man.

However, the very recent natural history of aluminum is concerning, and it marks the advent of what I have called "the Aluminum Age."[4] When, in 1889, Charles Martin Hall invented a process of extracting aluminum metal from its ubiquitous ores of the Earth's crust, it heralded an age as important as any before or since.[5] Aluminum metal and its many salts and myriad compounds were catalysts (both literally and metaphorically) for technological change fueling (again quite literally) the advances of the twentieth century and beyond. Aluminum was lauded as a miracle metal, and, as it eventually transpired, there were no limits to its applications in modern life and living. Throughout the seemingly infinitely long period when there has been life on Earth, human beings, in only the latter part of the nineteenth century, achieved something not seen before in Nature. We have presided over an ubiquitome of biologically reactive aluminum. I just made up the word *ubiquitome* to describe and to bring to life the biological world of aluminum (since aluminum is both omnipresent and biologically available, while only the former was true prior to the Aluminum Age). A Pandora's box of possibilities is open, and over a century of the consequences are already upon us. In the short term, at least, biologically reactive aluminum is only toxic, and its ubiquitome is why we should all worry about aluminum.

---

4 Exley, "The Aluminium Age," *The Hippocratic Post*, https://www.hippocraticpost.com/mens -health/the-aluminium-age/.

5 "Production of Aluminum: The Hall-Héroult Process," National Historic Chemical Landmark, Dedicated September 17, 1997 at Oberlin College in Oberlin, Ohio, and November 2, 2001 at Alcoa Inc., in Pittsburgh, Pennsylvania, https://www.acs.org/content/acs/en/education /whatischemistry/landmarks/aluminumprocess.html.

CHAPTER 3

Some Simple Aluminum Biochemistry

What do I mean when I write about biologically reactive aluminum? A brief introduction to the biological chemistry of aluminum should help to make this clearer. Stay with me: I know that just the word "chemistry" is an anathema to many and is often used as an excuse not to understand something. As a biologist (and not a chemist, as someone has reported on Wikipedia), I appreciated very early in my scientific career that I needed to understand chemistry, but primarily that I needed to understand *certain* chemistry. In my example, what I needed to know was the chemistry of aluminum as it impacts living things. Aluminum chemistry can be as complicated as it is ubiquitous. A one-thousand-page tome would almost certainly not do justice to the chemistry of this wonder metal. However, the aluminum that we have already described herein as biologically reactive has one distinct chemical form, and it is the solvated free metal cation (a positively charged ion), written as $Al^{3+}_{(aq)}$.[1] (The subscript "aq" stands for aqueous, so this tells us that Al^{3+} is the form of aluminum that is found in water, an aqueous solvent.) This is the form of aluminum bound by biological molecules in bringing about aluminum's toxicity. It may not be the only form to be biologically reactive. However, we know unequivocally that $Al^{3+}_{(aq)}$ is biologically reactive, and this certainty provides a solid baseline for understanding how aluminum influences biological processes and exerts its toxicity.

1 Christopher Exley, "Elucidating Aluminiums Exposome," *Current Inorganic Chemistry* 2, no. 1 (2012): 3–7, http://www.eurekaselect.com/96212/article?trendmd-shared=3.

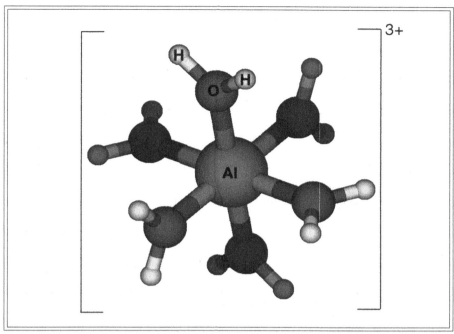

Figure 3. A model of biologically reactive aluminum. The aluminum atom is surrounded by six water molecules, giving an overall molecular charge of +3. *Courtesy of X. Lopez.* (See color version in insert.)

When $Al^{3+}_{(aq)}$ is bound by a biological molecule, for example a protein, this can be considered as aberrant, an unwanted interaction, since no biological molecule (or biomolecule) requires aluminum to be functional. Indeed, the opposite is usually the case, as binding aluminum, instead of an essential metal ion such as magnesium, renders the biomolecule dis- or nonfunctional. It no longer works as it is meant to work. Imagine biochemical systems as orchestras where essential metals such as magnesium are the conductors. The natural selection of the elements of life, a term coined by the father of bioinorganic chemistry, the late, great RJP Williams FRS, has ensured a faultless symphony. It is not then so difficult to envisage the ensuing cacophony when aluminum substitutes for an essential metal and, acting as conductor, directs notes from compromised instruments at all the wrong times. This perhaps overly poetic analogy reminds me of a famous exchange between the English comedian Eric Morecambe and German-American musician André Previn. The latter chastises the former for playing the wrong notes on a piano. Morecambe replies that he is actually playing all the right notes but in the wrong order! This is the biological chemistry of aluminum, and it is inevitably toxic.

Certain properties of a biomolecule make it an attractive partner for aluminum. When considering if a biomolecule will bind aluminum, an important factor is the availability of oxygen-based groups, such as phosphate on adenosine triphosphate (ATP) or carboxylic acid on citrate (citric acid), as these types of "functional groups" bind aluminum ($Al^{3+}_{(aq)}$) with avidity, forming strong and stable complexes. Oxygen-based groups, such as just described, are arguably the most common groups on biomolecules for binding metals in all biological systems, and this commonality underlies the preeminent toxicity of aluminum. Because of this propensity to be bound by common functional groups on myriad biomolecules, aluminum is uniquely positioned as an almost universal (disruptive) metal cofactor throughout biochemistry. However, like swallows and summer, as the saying goes, one strong aluminum-biomolecule complex doth not (well, rarely) overt toxicity make. Instead, biology is inherently robust, and before aluminum is toxic, it must overcome the resilience of any affected biochemistry or biological process. Toxicity is the result of many $Al^{3+}_{(aq)}$ being bound by equally numerous biomolecules within a relatively short period of time. Aluminum must overcome the defenses and storm the battlements before any toxicity ensues.[2]

By identifying $Al^{3+}_{(aq)}$ as the perpetrator of toxicity, all other forms of aluminum can be considered as sources of $Al^{3+}_{(aq)}$. All forms of aluminum, including metallic forms, will break down under certain conditions to release $Al^{3+}_{(aq)}$ for binding by biomolecules. This is a basic tenet underlying all understanding of the toxicity of aluminum in living things. Ask the question if any particular form of aluminum has the propensity to release significant quantities of $Al^{3+}_{(aq)}$. Those forms of aluminum that find themselves in a physiological compartment—an example of which would be blood—that promotes their rapid dissolution to produce a continuous supply of $Al^{3+}_{(aq)}$ are more likely to result in toxicity than other forms of aluminum in the same compartment, but that are less prone to breakdown. The availability of biologically reactive aluminum is governed by processes akin to Darwinian natural selection, with the environment (where the aluminum is found) playing a crucial role in any outcome. All of the aluminum found in, or associated with, the human body has the potential to result in toxicity.

2 Christopher Exley, "The toxicity of aluminium in humans/La toxicité de l'aluminium chez l'homme," *Morphologie* 100, no. 329 (June 2016): 51–55, https://www.sciencedirect.com /science/article/abs/pii/S1286011516000023.

Fulfilment of this potential leads to human disease. This is arguably all the basic chemistry required to have insight into the toxicity of aluminum, whether fish, fowl, or human being.[3]

3 Christopher Exley and Matthew J.Mold, "The binding, transport and fate of aluminium in biological cells," *Journal of Trace Elements in Medicine and Biology* 30 (April 2015): 90–95, https://www.sciencedirect.com/science/article/pii/S0946672X14002107?via%3Dihub.

CHAPTER 4

Where Is Aluminum in the Body?

We, my research group, have defined something that we call "the body burden of aluminum."[1] It is all of the aluminum that is associated with the body at any one time. It includes all of the aluminum that is on the inside of the body and, critically, all of the aluminum that is on the outside of the body. Aluminum that is on the inside must have passed through the body's outer surfaces, including the skin, the gut, the nose, and the lungs to reside eventually within body tissues. In comparison, aluminum that is on the outside of the body may be in the process of entering the body or it may be lodged, trapped, or caught within external surfaces, such as those of the skin, the gut, the lungs, and the nose.

While everyone can more easily acknowledge how diet contributes to the body burden of aluminum, it is perhaps not as well appreciated that topical applications of products that contain aluminum, including cosmetics, sunscreens, and antiperspirants, also add to the body burden of aluminum upon every application. For example, normal use of an aluminum-based antiperspirant might add as much as 1g of aluminum to the skin surface each day, while a day on the beach could involve applying as much as 5g of aluminum in sunscreen. All forms of aluminum associated with the body have the possibility to break down through disaggregation and dissolution and thereby release biologically reactive aluminum ($Al^{3+}_{(aq)}$). As such, they

1 Christopher Exley, "Human exposure to aluminium," *Environmental Science: Processes & Impacts* 10 (2013) https://pubs.rsc.org/en/content/articlelanding/2013/EM/C3EM00374D #!divAbstract.

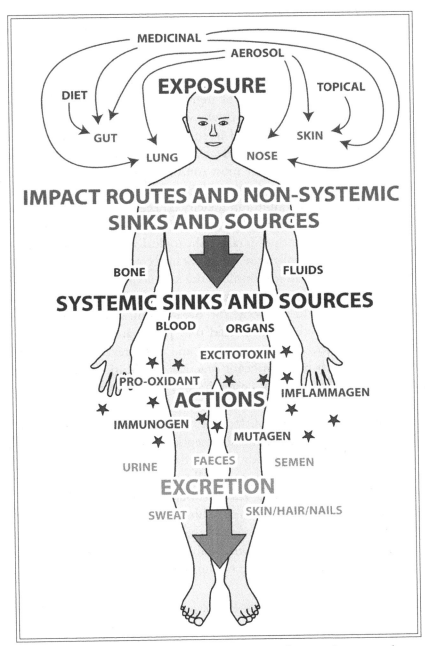

Figure 4. The schematic identifies the main factors, from uptake to excretion, involved with human exposure to aluminum. Please see the full paper for a complete explanation.** (See color version in insert.)

** Ibid.

must all be included in the body burden of aluminum. While aluminum associated with the outer surfaces of the body in time may enter the body, it also may exert toxicity without entering the body. Personally, I continue to worry about the promotion of sunscreen and sunblock, many versions of which include aluminum salts as ingredients. Aluminum is a powerful catalyst of oxidative damage (this is why we call it a pro-oxidant[2]) and with sunlight and the UV filters found in sunscreen, it forms a dangerous triumvirate capable of carcinogenic effects. Is it only a coincidence that those countries in the world using the most sunscreen per head have the highest incidence of melanoma?[3]

Another example of aluminum toxicity on the outside of the body is its inhibition of the activity of sweat glands in the skin through the application of an aluminum-based antiperspirant.[4] The topically applied aluminum salt, usually aluminum chlorohydrate, dissolves in secretions at the skin surface to release $Al^{3+}_{(aq)}$, which in turn inhibits the release of sweat by sweat glands. This is how an antiperspirant works, by affecting the activity of a major and important gland in the body, the sweat gland. The manufacturers of antiperspirants know this, but instead they propagate the myth that they work by simply blocking the sweat gland and thus preventing the secretion of sweat. This myth has significant practical implications, since it allows antiperspirants to be classed as cosmetics and not as medicine, thereby preventing unwieldy (for the manufacturers) regulation of their use.

The majority of the outer surfaces of the body, in terms of their surface area, is actually inside the body, the exception being the skin. These outer surfaces on the inside of the body, such as those in the gut and in the lung, are living, reactive surfaces and are equally prone to the disruptive effect of biologically reactive aluminum. The distribution of the body burden of aluminum is, at best, uncertain. There are historical data purporting to report aluminum content in tissues throughout the body. These data are, in general, from disparate sources of unknown reliability and cannot give an accurate understanding of the body burden of aluminum. Until the discrepancies in

2 Christopher Exley, "The pro-oxidant activity of aluminum," *Free Radical Biology and Medicine* 36, no. 3 (February 2004): 380–387, https://www.sciencedirect.com/science/article/abs/pii/S0891584903007937?via%3Dihub.

3 "Melanoma of the skin statistics," Australian Government, https://melanoma.canceraustralia.gov.au/statistics.

4 Christopher Exley, "Aluminum in antiperspirants: More than just skin deep," *The American Journal of Medicine* 117, no. 12 (December 15, 2004): 969–970, https://www.amjmed.com/article/S0002-9343(04)00694-1/fulltext.

these historical data are addressed in research designed specifically for the purpose of measuring the body burden of aluminum, certain assumptions are needed in answering the question: where is aluminum in the body? For example, long-lived body compartments have a greater propensity to accumulate aluminum over time. Bone is one such compartment. Growing bone presents a highly phosphorylated environment to innervating biological fluids, ostensibly to bind calcium but also highly attractive to biologically reactive aluminum. It is bound at the bone front and becomes trapped in growing bone, leaving an aluminum-rich area almost akin to the growth rings of a tree. The presence of an aluminum-rich area is a testimony to a time when an individual was experiencing a higher than usual exposure to aluminum.

It is also the case in aging and other circumstances of bone loss and bone remodeling that this "aluminum front" can become a source of biologically reactive aluminum to the rest of the body. Neurones, the brain cells, are the longest-lived cells in the body, and this makes them a prime target for the accumulation of aluminum over time.[5] The brain, like bone, is therefore a tissue in the body where you might expect to find aluminum. This longevity of neurones also makes them prime targets of aluminum toxicity, as toxic thresholds are reached over (usually) decades of continuous low exposure. Compare the latter to a skin cell that may live for only a few days or weeks. Skin cells in general are unlikely to suffer aluminum toxicity before being shed from the body. Exfoliation is one of the adventitious ways that aluminum is excreted or shed from the body. Other reservoirs of aluminum, potentially in transit, will be the lungs and the gut. Both of these major organs will house aluminum at their external surfaces and within their tissues. In many ways, these two organs are significant sources of aluminum with their individual burdens being in continuous exchange with other areas of the body. Other principal organs where one might expect to find aluminum are the liver and the kidney. Both are important in the excretion of aluminum, again adventitious, from the body, the liver via the bile and the gut and the kidney with urine.

5 Christopher Exley, "Why industry propaganda and political interference cannot disguise the inevitable role played by human exposure to aluminum in neurodegenerative diseases, including Alzheimer's disease," *Frontiers in Neurology* 27 (October 2014) https://www .frontiersin.org/articles/10.3389/fneur.2014.00212/full.

CHAPTER 5

Measuring the Body Burden of Aluminum

There is a burgeoning trend for individuals to want to measure what is in their body, and aluminum is no exception to this. Often people are hoping to self-diagnose a suspected intoxication by aluminum, and, following the latest trend in "detox," they want to know if the treatment has reduced their body burden of aluminum. This is completely understandable as is the concomitant advent of burgeoning commercial outlets offering tests for aluminum on a variety of biological indices, including blood, urine, and hair. The latter is the most widely available test and a popular choice due to ease of applicability. However, what scrutiny is given to the value of the data obtained or provided from these tests? Often somewhere between very little and none. The precise and reliable determination of aluminum in any tissue of the body is notoriously difficult for a plethora of very good reasons. In my laboratory, we have spent over thirty years optimizing our methods, and even our data on aluminum cannot always be beyond criticism. This fact alone should act as a warning that commercial outlets advertising measurement of aluminum in human tissues cannot provide reliable and reproducible data. Until the time that this is possible, everyone would be better advised to save their money. However, if there were opportunities to obtain precise, reliable, and robust measurements of aluminum through certified laboratories using standard methods, then what might be learned from the measurement of aluminum in hair, blood, and urine?

Let's Start with Hair

Perhaps hair is the most problematic of these tissues, as an assumption is always made that the source of aluminum in hair is the systemic circulation. However, is this really the case? What about contamination of hair from the external environment, including dyes, shampoos, conditioners, and other hair care products? The success of these products often involves their active ingredient being bound tightly to hair; and, in the case of some, for example many dyes, aluminum may actually be the linking agent added for this purpose. Aluminum in these products applied to hair will be extremely difficult to remove and will result in erroneously high data for hair aluminum content. Assuming hair can be clean with no extraneous contamination, then the aluminum content in hair is usually further interpreted as a surrogate for aluminum in blood. Therefore, the assumption follows that aluminum present in blood nurturing growing hair is deposited at the growth front. As hair grows, aluminum remains trapped in the protein, mainly keratin, the matrix of the hair, even after the hair has died. The aluminum content of hair can then be measured accurately. However, what would the subsequent data indicate about the body burden of aluminum? What would it tell you about your personal exposure to aluminum? Does a high content of hair aluminum indicate similar quantities in the blood or, perhaps, does it indicate a slow build-up or accumulation of aluminum over a particular time?

To begin to be useful, measurements of hair aluminum require strict control conditions. It may be helpful to examine such conditions; for example, how should we go about taking hair samples for subsequent analysis of their aluminum content? Let us consider a hair analysis protocol that just might provide useful data relating to the body burden of aluminum:

1. Begin by designating an area of hair growth on the body. For example, the nape of the neck.
2. Shave the hair from this area, making sure to avoid any unnecessary abrasion of the skin surface.
3. Clean the designated area with a solvent known to be free of contamination by aluminum. Ultrapure water may be the best choice, as otherwise how would you know if the solvent was aluminum-free without actually having to measure it?
4. Allow hair in the designated area to regrow to a predetermined length while during this period ensuring that no cleaning solutions

other than the original aluminum-free solvent are applied to the hair.

5. Harvest all hair from the designated area, again ensuring that no skin is removed or any abrasions to the skin are incurred. Use sterile stainless steel scissors or clippers.

6. Ensure that a minimum weight of hair (e.g., 100 mg) is available for microwave-assisted acid/peroxide digestion. The hair must be converted to a solution.

7. Measure total content of aluminum in the solution obtained from the weighed hair sample using either TH GFAAS or ICP MS.

8. Finally, compare the data achieved with a database of reference values.

At this point readers will, I hope, appreciate that obtaining valuable information on an individual's body burden of aluminum from hair analyses is not a trivial task and that the method just described herein in its simplest form cannot be achieved by and is not reproduced in tests provided by commercial outlets. Hair analyses, performed outside of the very best academic research laboratories, are not yet reliable biological indicators of the body burden of aluminum.

What About Blood?

The use of blood as an estimate of exposure to aluminum is also problematic. While hair samples can in theory be taken by anyone, only qualified skilled clinicians should take blood samples. When a sample of blood is taken, there is neither evidence nor reason to believe that, at the time of sampling, aluminum will be homogeneously distributed throughout the whole blood volume of an individual.[1] Whole blood is a tissue, and it includes many different compartments. Blood is a heterogeneous mixture that acts throughout the body. One sample of blood taken from a particular vessel is only a moment in time and space; it cannot accurately reflect the aluminum concentration in the whole blood volume, never mind thereafter be further interpreted in respect of the aluminum content in tissues. It is a snapshot; if it shows a high value, then this might be a cause for concern; but

1 Christopher Exley, James Beardmore, and Gordon Rugg, "Computational approach to the blood–aluminum problem?" *International Journal of Quantum Chemistry* 107, no. 2 (2007): 275–278, https://onlinelibrary.wiley.com/doi/abs/10.1002/qua.21190.

if it gives a low value, this should not be interpreted as a low body burden of aluminum. Multiple, timed blood samples over a specified period, such as twenty-four hours, would be more informative, though such are rarely attempted and also carry with them multiple dangers that are always inherent in blood sampling. Once blood has been taken, there is then the question of how it will be processed and whether to use whole blood, plasma, or serum in any subsequent analyses. These issues with blood sampling are considerations that are rarely, if ever, addressed by those using blood as an indicator of the body burden of aluminum. One additional problem that is not always appreciated is that some ready-to-use syringes for sampling blood include constituents that are aluminum-based, such as coagulants, or may be contaminated with aluminum. Unfortunately, the peer-reviewed scientific literature is awash with data on blood aluminum where these issues of contamination had not been anticipated. I am only guessing, but these problems are almost certainly even more acute in commercial sampling and measurement of aluminum in blood.

Routine analyses of hair and blood do not yet tell us what we want to know. The resulting data are insufficient in themselves as indicators of reliable estimates of how much aluminum is in the body. In addition, they tell us almost nothing about aluminum associated with the outer surfaces of the body. However, if an assumption were made that all aluminum inside the body (systemic aluminum) can be represented as an equilibrium between the tissues and body fluids, primarily blood, then data representing blood aluminum over an extended time would be a useful estimate of the internal body burden. The latter, though incomplete, is still preferable to no estimate at all of the body burden of aluminum.

We Advocate Urine

In my laboratory, we consider urinary excretion of aluminum the best relative biological indicator of an individual's lifetime exposure to aluminum, the latter being the balance between all forms of exposure and all consequences of its removal from the body. The formation of urine involves the filtration of blood over time and is a continuous process. The kidney essentially "samples" the blood, removing from it all forms of aluminum that are below a critical size. The glomerulus of the kidney is its filter and is permeable to all forms and complexes of aluminum that have a molecular weight below 18000 Daltons. Note that this molecular weight excludes major blood proteins such as transferrin, the iron transport protein, and albumin, another transport protein. Both of these proteins, and especially transferrin, bind aluminum, and so they are not vehicles for the direct removal of aluminum from blood via the kidney. Aluminum collects in urine, which is then excreted from the body in discrete volumes during the day. Urine is what is described as a composite sample; it is an average of the aluminum content of the filterable fraction of blood (< 18000 Daltons MW, or molecular weight) over a specific time. Further assumptions are that the filterable fraction of aluminum in blood is in a dynamic equilibrium with both the rest of the blood—such as blood cells and higher molecular weight proteins—and body tissues. Which means that when aluminum is removed from the lower molecular weight fraction of the blood by the kidney, it is subsequently immediately replaced, even replenished, by aluminum moving from other compartments such as the tissues. This is what is meant by a dynamic equilibrium. Because urine is processed and excreted over time, it accommodates, or takes into account, one of the main criticisms of taking blood samples, that being the temporal nature of the concentration of aluminum in blood. While a blood sample is only representative of a time and place when blood is taken, a urine sample reflects blood aluminum throughout the body and over an extended period. Arguably, the most useful urine samples are those where all urine produced in a twenty-four-hour period is collected. By measuring both the aluminum content of such a composite sample and the total urine volume during this period, urinary aluminum excretion can be expressed as a weight of aluminum in twenty-four hours. It gives information on how much aluminum is excreted in a specific twenty-four-hour period. If, for ethical reasons or simply because of convenience, only "spot" samples of urine can be taken, for example just a single sample or a sample every so often, then any analysis of aluminum content must be normalized against dilution of the urine. To explain, when urine is made in the kidney, water is reabsorbed from the urine, making it a concentrated product to be stored in the bladder. The reabsorption of water from urine in the kidney is not a constant, and readers will be well aware of those personal circumstances when their urine is more dilute or more concentrated than usual. For example, certain products, such as alcohol, inhibit the antidiuretic hormone and reduce the absorption of water from urine, resulting in a dilute urine. Aluminum is not reabsorbed along with water and neither is something called creatinine (a breakdown product from muscle that passes from the blood to the urine), and so for spot measurements of aluminum in urine, the aluminum content is expressed as a weight of aluminum per weight of creatinine. Data on urinary excretion of aluminum, expressed either per twenty-four hours or per unit of creatinine, have proven useful and reliable relative estimates of the body burden of aluminum. Ideally, the nature of any body burden is confirmed using urine samples collected over five consecutive days. While this might be considered as burdensome, taking urine samples does not have the same issues as either blood or hair, and the data are eminently more reliable. The following is an example of a protocol used in my laboratories.

Urine Sampling to Estimate the Body Burden of Aluminum

We use urinary excretion of aluminum over two consecutive days to establish if an individual has a higher than usual body burden of aluminum. This procedure should be organized with the participation of an individual's general practitioner or equivalent expert in health. They should have access to all the necessary sampling materials as required, as well as knowledge of certified laboratories where urine analyses can be carried out. We provide advice on all of these procedures if required.

Results should be presented as μmoles (or μg) Al excreted per 24h and μmoles Al / μmole creatinine. We can advise on whether or not the values obtained are significantly different from those that would be considered normal for someone of the same gender and age.

The protocol is carried out over an initial period of two consecutive days:

Day 1—Participants provide a twenty-four-hour urine sample while following their regular diet. This acts as a control sample. Thus, all urine produced during a preset period of twenty-four hours is collected into a single vessel.

Day 2—Participants provide a second twenty-four-hour urine sample after drinking up to 1.5L of a silicon-rich mineral water.[2] The mineral water should, if possible, be drunk at regular intervals throughout the waking day. The participant is free to continue with their regular daily diet as normal. As per day one, all urine produced during this second period of twenty-four hours is collected into a single vessel.

---

2 A silicon-rich mineral water is defined as any commercially available mineral water where the natural content of silicon (expressed as silica) exceeds 30 mg/L or ppm.

Urine samples should be collected into pristine twenty-four-hour urine containers (these are made-for-purpose containers that should be available through the general practitioner or equivalent). If possible, the participant should store urine samples in biohazard bags in their refrigerator before they are delivered to or picked up by their clinic or laboratory. Participants should be provided with a plastic pristine sample jug for ease of urine collection. It is extremely important that all urine be collected so that a final urine volume per twenty-four hours can be determined. Do not attempt to wash the jug between urine samples, as this could introduce contamination.

Urine samples, one from each day, should be analyzed for total aluminum. Total creatinine should also be measured. We provide advice on methodology if required. By comparing urinary excretion on day one with that of day two, we can get an understanding if an individual may be experiencing an overload of aluminum. To confirm an aluminum overload, we would recommend that the same protocol be carried out, not over two consecutive days, but over two consecutive periods of five days. Thus, five days without drinking a silicon-rich mineral water followed by five days while drinking a silicon-rich mineral water.

I hope that by providing you with all this detailed information it will be clear that, in reality in 2020, unless you have access to state-of-the-art laboratory facilities and the commensurate expertise, accurate and useful measurements of aluminum in the body are impossible. This situation can improve, especially if laboratories that offer these services adopt practices that are more robust and are based upon the latest published scientific research. One approach, to be pursued first in an academic environment, is to relate rigorous data from two distinct sampling methods. For example, we could compare per individual data on aluminum in hair with that for urinary excretion. Positive correlations would begin to validate hair as a biological indicator for everyday exposure to aluminum. Until we can be better assured about methods and meaning of data, my advice is to save your money and not pay for commercial tests relating to how much aluminum is in the human body.

CHAPTER 6

Aluminum In Doesn't Equal Aluminum Out

Accepting that we cannot accurately know our individual body burdens of aluminum, understanding human exposure to aluminum needs some practical everyday rules: specifically, how to reduce intake and increase removal. Currently, all evidence that originates from measurements of human biopsy tissue points toward accumulation of aluminum in the body with age. A proviso is that this rule only seems to hold true for neurologically unimpaired individuals[1] and also becomes less significant in older age.[2] Paradoxically, healthy people accumulate aluminum in the body with age, and this relationship only falls down once you become unhealthy, due to aluminum or otherwise. Nevertheless, a regime is needed to reverse this trend, something that might be easier said than done in the Aluminum Age.

Aluminum in the environment associates with every outer surface of the body, and these same surfaces are routes of uptake of aluminum into the body. One such surface is the skin, with its varied physical and chemical

---

1 C. Linhart, D. Davidson, S. Pathmanathan, T. Kamaladas, and C. Exley, "Aluminium in Brain Tissue in Non-neurodegenerative/Non-neurodevelopmental Disease: A Comparison with Multiple Sclerosis," *Exposure and Health* (2020) https://link.springer.com/article/10.1007/s12403-020-00346-9#Sec6.

2 Christopher Exley and Elizabeth Clarkson, "Aluminium in human brain tissue from donors without neurodegenerative disease: A comparison with Alzheimer's disease, multiple sclerosis and autism," *Scientific Reports* 10 (May 8, 2020) https://www.nature.com/articles/s41598-020-64734-6.

properties. Contrary to popular understanding, skin is permeable to aluminum, and it supports points of entry at levels that are macroscopic, such as pores leading to sweat glands, and those that are microscopic, including structural components that allow the passage of nanoparticles and fat-loving organics, the latter of which dissolves into the skin surface. Research on the permeability of skin to aluminum in living humans (as opposed to excised patches of skin) is almost nonexistent. There are no reliable quantitative data. For example, how much aluminum is absorbed across the skin when the body is immersed in a solution of aluminum? When you take a bath is an example. The usual assumption is that absorption is negligible, but this is simply unknown, and only future research will help to answer this and similar questions. A few years ago, I collaborated with a Polish geochemist, and we investigated silicon and aluminum chemistry in a large number of curative waters in Poland.[3] These are waters renowned for their health benefits, similar to spa waters in other countries. We did find that a significant number of them were rich in soluble silicon—silicic acid—and, as I will write about later herein, this raised the specter of this property being the background to the reported health benefits of these waters. Unfortunately, we never were able to perform the obvious follow-up research to establish if bathing in water that was rich in silicic acid resulted in its increased concentration in the blood. Just perhaps was it these curative waters, found throughout Europe, that Louis Pasteur had in mind when he is reported to have said, "Effects of silicic acid are destined to play a great and major role in therapy"? Great man that he was, he may, of course, have made the mistake that many make in confusing silicic acid with salicylic acid (aspirin)! A slip of the tongue, no less.

Actually, a paucity of reliable research is the conclusion most often reached when the "permeability" (how much gets in) of the human body to aluminum is questioned. Current understanding is mainly informed by dogma, the classic example of which concerns the question of how much ingested aluminum is absorbed across the gut.[4] There are major discrep-

---

3 Dariusz Dobrzynski and Christopher Exley, "Solubility control and therapeutic potential of silicon in curative mineral waters of the Sudetes Mountains, Poland," *Acta Balneologica* 52 (January 2010) https://www.researchgate.net/profile/Dariusz_Dobrzynski2 /publication/235889891_Solubility_control_and_therapeutic_potential_of_silicon_in_curative _mineral_waters_of_the_Sudetes_Mountains_Poland/links/09e41513df7e2d3c97000000 /Solubility-control-and-therapeutic-potential-of-silicon-in-curative-mineral-waters-of-the-Sudetes -Mountains-Poland.pdf.

4 Christopher Exley, "Human exposure to aluminium," *Environmental Science: Processes & Impacts*, https://pubs.rsc.org/en/content/articlelanding/2013/EM/C3EM00374D#!divAbstract.

ancies in the available data, depending, for example, on the design of the experiment. Research measuring the occurrence of aluminum in the bloodstream, usually the hepatic portal vein, following its ingestion in a variety of guises usually estimates the percentage of absorption as anything between 0.1 and 1 percent. However, by way of contrast, research measuring the aluminum content of stools (feces, not a popular experiment) following ingestion of aluminum can only account for 70 percent of ingested aluminum. It is assumed that the remaining 30 percent is absorbed across the gut or perhaps retained within the architecture of the gut. We are left with an estimate for the absorption of aluminum across the gut of between 0.1 and 30 percent and the three hundredfold difference is probably an accurate reflection of a true range based upon the myriad forms in which aluminum is ingested and differences in gut physiology between individuals. It is generally accepted that a significant proportion of individuals, perhaps 10 percent, are superabsorbers of aluminum across the gut. Such predictions originate from healthy volunteer studies where absorption is estimated from the concentration of aluminum in hepatic portal vein blood following ingestion of an aluminum-containing drink on an empty stomach. Therefore, the data are prone to the vagaries already identified, but, nominally at least, they do suggest that absorption of aluminum across the gut is subject to individual differences in human physiology. We do not know why some individuals absorb significantly more aluminum. However, research involving individuals with certain genetic predispositions leading to Down's syndrome and familial Alzheimer's disease does suggest a possible genetic origin. It is intriguing to speculate that genetic diversity within human populations, such as is seen in conditions like autism or Alzheimer's disease, predisposes individuals to a higher body burden of aluminum and that this genetic diversity may not lead to such disease in the absence of aluminum. There will be more on this later. Another important surface that must be involved in the entry of aluminum into the body is the lungs. The huge surface area of the lungs presents significant opportunities for the absorption of aluminum as well as for trapping airborne aluminum. The latter may eventually end up in the gut through efficient and continuous cleaning of lung surfaces by secretion of mucus, the same substance that, in a more dilute form, makes up saliva in the mouth. Therefore, the gut receives aluminum in the diet and additionally from the air as aluminum that has been trapped in the lungs and transported to the gut. The internal surfaces of the mouth should not be ignored as vehicles for the uptake of aluminum into the body. Sublingual (under the tongue) and buccal (between gums and cheek) surfaces are often employed as routes of administration of drugs to improve their uptake into the blood. The same logic applies to them as surfaces for the absorption of aluminum, though, to my knowledge, this remains to be confirmed experimentally for aluminum. Another surface that is well known as a rapid uptake route for drugs is the olfactory epithelium accessed via the nasal cavity. It is not a coincidence that a number of social drugs, including cocaine, are taken through the nose. Passage via the olfactory route offers direct access to the hippocampus in the brain, and this is a likely route of entry for aluminum into brain tissue. An example of which is exposure to particulate aluminum in the workplace leading to Alzheimer's disease.[5]

The opportunities for aluminum to enter the human body are manifold. Some researchers try to quantify these opportunities through modeling and similar methods and look thereby to provide estimates of human exposure to aluminum. While laudable objectives, the knowledge and data currently available are not sufficient for these practices to be any more than academic tasks. Of course, such exposure limits are primary whims of policy-forming agencies where science is not the only important criterion. The results of these efforts may often fool reviewers and editors alike and enter the pub-lished record, but they cannot have any real-life meaning and inevitably only further mislead all on this subject. Research on living human beings is difficult and, rightly, tightly controlled. However, it is worth asking the question as to how we know that in a living person aluminum crosses all of the aforementioned surfaces or barriers and enters the body. How do we know that there is at least one atom of aluminum in every cell, in every compartment of the body? Well, we know that there is aluminum in the body because we can measure its presence in waste products originating from inside the body. However, the presence of aluminum in excreta, secre-tions, and shed tissues is entirely adventitious. It is there through accidents of chemistry, and its measurement confirms not only that aluminum enters the body, but that it leaves the body, too.

The stool (feces) is probably the body's excretion richest in aluminum, though the assumption is that most fecal aluminum originates from undi-gested food. However, some aluminum in feces will come from inside the body, having been removed from the blood by the liver, thereafter to be

5 Christopher Exley and Thomas Vickers, "Elevated brain aluminium and early onset Alzheimer's disease in an individual occupationally exposed to aluminium: a case report," *Journal of Medical Case Reports* 8 (2014) https://jmedicalcasereports.biomedcentral.com /articles/10.1186/1752-1947-8-41.

excreted into the gut in bile. The kidney also passively filters aluminum from the blood, and urinary excretion may represent the main route of departure of aluminum from the body. Recent data now implicate perspiration as a significant route whereby aluminum leaves the body. How aluminum accumulates in sweat is unknown, but individuals can perspire up to four liters of sweat in a single day, which puts sweating perhaps on an equal footing with urinary excretion with respect to its importance in removing aluminum from the body.[6] Other secretions known to contain significant amounts of aluminum include breast milk, semen, and sebum. We also lose aluminum with our hair, our nails, and our skin, all through natural or aggravated shedding.

Manifold routes of departure match manifold routes of entry of aluminum into the body. This area of human exposure to aluminum research is calling out for whole-body, climate-controlled experiments. In an example, participants live in a climate-controlled environment for a specific time during which the aluminum content of everything that they eat, use, or apply is measured along with the aluminum content of breathed air. All excreta, secretions, and, where possible, shed tissues produced during the specific time are collected and their aluminum content measured. Data obtained would allow some sort of mass balance between aluminum in and aluminum out to be calculated. Of course, the suggested experiments are impractical, as it would be difficult to recruit participants to take part for more than a few days. In addition, the data would have many provisos and assumptions, but, for the specific period of the study, they would still represent the most informative data in this area yet obtained for living people. We would have the first complete and arguably informative data on whether aluminum in equals aluminum out or not.

---

6 Clare Minshall, Jodie Nadal, and Christopher Exley, "Aluminium in human sweat," *Journal of Trace Elements in Medicine and Biology* 28, no. 1 (January 2014): 87–88, https://www .sciencedirect.com/science/article/abs/pii/S0946672X13001612.

CHAPTER 7

I Am the Aluminum I Eat (or Am I?)

Diet, food, drink, and sundry supplements are perhaps obvious ways in which we are exposed to aluminum. However, what are the dietary practices that really make a difference in how much aluminum enters the gut? What is it about one diet that exposes an individual to more or less aluminum on a daily basis? Is it the amount of aluminum in the diet that is important, or is it the amount that is retained in tissues? I cannot give specific answers to these questions, but I can provide some helpful guidance.

There have been a number of detailed studies aiming to establish the aluminum content of whole diets. The idea behind these studies seems to be to estimate how much aluminum an individual consumes in food and drink on a daily basis. These appear to be mainly nation-specific in that I am aware of similar studies estimating dietary aluminum in Chinese, Spanish, Italian, French, German, and American populations. The aluminum content of food groups, derived from measurements of aluminum in myriad products, estimates how much aluminum is in idealized everyday diets. By design, the studies conclude with average data for average individuals in an average country. Subsequently, there is always, apparently, a need to compare these quantitative data with some form of regulatory—well, in reality, they are advisory—standard. The latter, for example produced by organizations such as the Food and Drugs Administration (FDA), European Food Standards Agency (EFSA), or the Food and Agriculture Organization (FAO), assume significant importance with respect to whether or not their suggested safety limits are exceeded by the average diet or not. Yes, there are arbitrary, recommended, nonenforceable safety limits for aluminum (that benign benefactor) in the diet. For example, many glibly cite EFSA's tolerable safety limit of 1 mg aluminum per kg of body weight per week, as if this criterion were an established scientific fact. As if it were a safety limit that would help to protect against the toxicity of ingested aluminum. Almost no one—scientists, policy makers, or otherwise—citing this (in)tolerable weekly limit (TWI) has investigated its origin. If they did, they would find that it is based upon very few scientific studies on animals—yes, on animals—not humans. As the Elephant Man, John Merrick, famously cried out to his assailants, "I am not an animal," and he is correct.

Please do not be deceived by these totally arbitrary limits relating to aluminum in diet. Their basis is not human consumption, and they have no relevance to human safety. They are not regulatory limits, and there is no human health-based legislation governing the aluminum content of food. The so-called scientists who sit on these various committees agreeing on these limits based upon the barest of evidence should be ashamed of themselves. Their participation, by design or through simple ignorance, in such charades can only serve as a smokescreen for complacency by industries and governments. The objective of such committees is clearly to ensure that much-needed actual research on human exposure to aluminum is not carried out. How many times have colluding authors concluded in their esteemed publications that exposure to aluminum through eating a particular food or diet does not exceed EFSA's, or some other recommended, limit? Too many times. It should be noted that the vast majority of studies looking at the aluminum content of whole diets, in particular, are carried out by state-sponsored organizations primarily looking to complete box-checking exercises. They are not really interested in the science of the subject, and they are certainly not concerned about understanding aluminum in diet and human health. These studies may have the appearance of legitimacy, but in-depth scrutiny of their content often reveals selected reference to the available scientific literature leading to purposefully ambiguous conclusions.[1]

If you are reading this book, then you are probably already health-aware and you understand the importance of diet in health. The only helpful research that I am aware of involving comparisons of whole diets

---

1 Thomas Tietz, Ariane Lenzner, Anna Elena Kolbaum, Sebastian Zellmer, Christian Riebeling, Rainer Gürtler, Christian Jung, Oliver Kappenstein, Jutta Tentschert, Michael Giulbudagian, Stefan Merkel, Ralph Pirow, Oliver Lindtner, Tewes Tralau, Bernd Schäfer, Peter Laux, Matthias Greiner, Alfonso Lampen, Andreas Luch, Reiner Wittkowski, and Andreas Hensel, "Aggregated aluminium exposure: risk assessment for the general population," *Archives of Toxicology* 93 (October 2019): 3503–3521, https://link.springer.com/article/10.1007/s00204-019-02599-z.

demonstrates that what has become known as "the Mediterranean diet" is significantly lower in aluminum content than a diet dominated by processed food and drink. I will expand upon this later in the book, but as a general rule of thumb, quality ingredients resourced respectfully and cooked at home (with love) will help you to lower your body burden of aluminum and to actually be something akin to what you eat.

CHAPTER 8

Live Safely and Effectively in the Aluminum Age

This is what it is all about. The Aluminum Age is upon us, and it is not going away anytime soon.[1] It is a mistake to believe that anyone other than yourself will protect you from aluminum. How can we manage everyday life to reduce our overall exposure to aluminum? How can we live safely and effectively in the Aluminum Age? I have been studying human exposure to aluminum for nearly forty years, and I know that it is simply not practical to believe that you can abstain completely from the Aluminum Age. To attempt to do so would diminish the quality of life to such an extent as to render it unlivable, if not unbearable. It would be something akin to the atrocities being committed by governments right now due to the tyranny of COVID-19. However, government tyranny aside, I am an optimist, and there are some changes in lifestyle that, if implemented, could make a difference. These are factors within our control.

Food and Drink

The most obvious and perhaps most easily adjusted are dietary factors, specifically in relation to our consumption of processed and unprocessed food and drink. I am using the term "processed" relatively liberally here

---

1 Christopher Exley, "The Aluminium Age," *The Hippocratic Post*, https://www.hippocraticpost .com/mens-health/the-aluminium-age/.

to mainly refer to convenience eating (i.e., fast food, ready-to-eat food, or simply complete meals that only require a few seconds in the microwave). Many food items have to undergo some form of processing before they are available to us, such as cured meats, and these would not necessarily fall under my definition of processed food.

Processed food and drink is always going to represent a higher overall dietary exposure to aluminum than unprocessed food and drink. There are a number of reasons for this, not the least of which being that aluminum salts are ingredients of processed food and drink. They are not included for their nutritional value since we know that they have none, but for their properties to (i) expedite processing of the product, (ii) facilitate point of use of the product, and (iii) improve the overall aesthetic qualities of the product. The addition of aluminum salts makes products cheaper to produce, easier for the customer to use, and more pleasant to the eye, i.e., overall a more attractive purchase. All of this is achieved at very little cost to manufacturers, as aluminum salts are extremely cheap in comparison to other ingredients and the final cost of the product to consumers. Classic examples include their addition to milk powders to prevent them from clumping and their incorporation in bread making to produce the iconic sliced white loaf, with aluminum sulfate being added as a whitener. There are myriad examples of these applications, and though the inclusion of aluminum salts and complexes is, or at least should be, written on the product packaging as a constituent, such is not always easy to recognize. For example, many E numbers (codes for substances used as food additives within the European Union) are actually aluminum compounds. One is left wondering if the invention of the use of E numbers was simply to disguise the addition of certain compounds to foods. Why not simply put the name of the additive in the list of ingredients on the packaging? In many ways the innumerable and burgeoning applications of aluminum salts in the processing of food is testimony, should it be needed, to the diverse chemistry of aluminum and why its advent heralded the Aluminum Age. Of course, the safety for humans of the myriad uses of aluminum in food should have been tested before this particular genie was released from the security of its geochemical, proverbial lamp.

The processing of food and drink necessarily involves substantial machinery and equipment and represents significant opportunities for contamination. Thus, aluminum enters products adventitiously as opposed to being an added ingredient for a particular purpose. Contamination by aluminum of processed food and drink is a major issue and usually only becomes known during routine monitoring by regulatory organizations or through the actions of individual enlightened scientists. As I write this, I am reminded of the great Bavarian pretzel scandal where high concentrations of aluminum in these traditional products were traced to the use of sodium hydroxide as a baste and aluminum metal cooking trays. Sodium hydroxide is highly alkaline and readily dissolves aluminum metal. The resulting aluminized pretzel is definitely more than most Bavarians were prepared to chew! It is a little sad that it takes an obscure example such as this for aluminum to make a news headline. Regulatory agencies such as the EFSA or the FDA are often reluctant to highlight these issues of contamination for fear of upsetting industry, often preferring to be (mis)guided by their own wayward standards. In the meantime, curious independent scientists can be more proactive, an example being my own group's research into the aluminum content of infant formulas. More on that scandal will come later in the book.

Processed food and drink is inevitably packaged, and if the product is in any way prone to oxidative damage, then the packaging housing the product will include aluminum. Next time you are browsing in your supermarket or local convenience store, notice how many different products are contained within foil-like packaging made of aluminum. The list of products is literally endless as new products protected by oxygen-resistant aluminum packaging arrive on the shelves every day. Packaging is a serious source of contamination of product by aluminum. Well-known examples are aluminum cans used for drinks and other liquids. When questioned about the safety of these cans, manufacturers will indicate that there is a layer, usually a plastic or polythene surface, between the aluminum metal and the stored product. This, they believe, is their "get out of jail free" card. However, what they choose not to tell you is that these protective layers always include flaws, and these bring the product into direct contact with the aluminum body of the can or container. Even if a product entering an aluminum can is devoid of aluminum, which, due to contamination during processing is already highly unlikely, it only requires a flaw in the inert inner surface of the can to allow the release of a fraction of a milligram of aluminum from the body of the can for that product to be significantly contaminated. Products stored in aluminum cans, such as many soft drinks, are themselves often of a chemical nature that will promote and accelerate the corrosion of aluminum, and this chemistry only adds to the inevitability of their contamination by aluminum. All independent peer-reviewed published research—and there is a great deal of it—confirms this contamination by aluminum cans and similar issues can be found in other forms of packaging that include an aluminum foil to prevent the ingress of oxygen, notably long-life Tetra Pak-style packaging.

May I digress with a related story? Late one morning, in Spring 2000 I believe, I received a telephone call from someone in a bar in Sydney, Australia. The caller identified himself as being the boss of a small sports drink company called Musashi. He explained to me that in their product advertising, they made a big deal out of not using packaging such as long-life Tetra Pak to avoid the possibility of contamination of their sports drinks by aluminum. Well, as you might imagine, Tetra Pak did not take kindly to this form of advertising and were taking Musashi to court, a process that could inevitably lead to bankruptcy for Musashi. I suggested that they send me all the science that Tetra Pak was relying upon to prove that their packaging did not contaminate products with aluminum. It did not take me long to use Tetra Pak's own internal product data, as supplied to me by Musashi, to prove that Tetra Pak was wrong. My first and, as yet only, trip to Australia saw me spend several days in the federal court without even being brought to the witness stand. Tetra Pak did not wish to risk putting me on the stand to defend my report. I am pleased to say that Musashi remains to this day a small, successful sports nutrition company. Tetra Pak on the other hand continues to use their aluminum-based packaging without any concessions toward its propensity to contaminate the products within. My advice is to avoid all products contained within long-life Tetra Pak packaging.

Processed foods and drinks are characterized by a higher content of aluminum, whether this is due to its being added as an ingredient, arriving adventitiously through processing, or being a contaminant from packaging. However, natural products can also contain significant amounts of aluminum, and this is usually a consequence of how and where they are grown. For example, many of the world's staple crops are grown intensively on acidic soils where the uptake of aluminum into the plant from the soil is expedited. Note that the soils are acidic because of poor agricultural practices, primarily related to intensification. Many such crops, including tea, coffee, and soya, tolerate aluminum in their tissues with the result being that their subsequent harvest and ingestion can represent significant dietary exposure to aluminum. None of these crops require aluminum for healthy growth. The opposite is true, and it is farming practices that have resulted in their contamination, primarily from soil, by aluminum; you might notice that this is similar to what happens in food processing.

Human activity is nearly always the reason why aluminum enters the living cycle. Arable crop farming may also be responsible for increased dietary exposure to aluminum through the extensive use of spray-on products, including herbicides, fungicides, and insecticides. Many such products either are aluminum-based compounds or include aluminum as a significant component. The widespread use of these products may be a significant contributor to recorded declines in populations of insect pollinators. Why else would the pupae of bumblebees be so heavily contaminated with aluminum?[2] As a brief aside, it is my belief that the current controversy concerning the herbicide glyphosate is in some way related to this compound's strong binding of aluminum at low pH, increasing the biological availability of aluminum in the human gut. Could glyphosate in "natural" products such as cereals, grains, and pulses be expediting the uptake of dietary aluminum across our gut? Our diet is an important component of everyday exposure to aluminum, and by reducing the proportion of processed products, you will lower your overall intake of aluminum in food and drink.

Medication

Medication is a significant and yet largely unquantified source of aluminum in the body. Many will be aware of the use of aluminum-based antacids for controlling reflux. These products have been the subject of both research and debate, although there can be no denying that they represent a very high exposure to aluminum. They are, to my knowledge, the only medication where the patient information leaflet warns against regular use to avoid development of neurological disease, including Alzheimer's disease. There is a stark example of Alzheimer's disease caused through prolonged use of antacids in Bert Ehgartner's outstanding documentary *The Age of Aluminum*.[3] This warning on the patient information leaflet that accompanies the drug is one of those equally rare situations where the pharmaceutical industry admits, in small print that almost no one reads, that aluminum is a probable cause of Alzheimer's disease while outwardly maintaining their official

---

2　Christopher Exley, Ellen Rotheray, and David Goulson, "Bumblebee Pupae Contain High Levels of Aluminium," *PLoS ONE* 10, no. 6 (June 4, 2015) https://journals.plos.org/plosone/article?id=10.1371/journal.pone.0127665.

3　"The Age of Aluminium (Die Akte Aluminium)," accessed September 30, 2020, https://www.youtube.com/watch?v=5F0u54gs0iU.

position that there is no link. This is an example of hedging your bets for insurance purposes if ever there was one.

A similar health warning should accompany the use of aluminum salts as phosphate binders in individuals undergoing kidney dialysis. While aluminum helps to reduce the absorption of phosphate from the gut, it is present to such an excess in these medications that its movement into the blood is inevitable, and its subsequent uptake into the brain is responsible for dialysis-related encephalopathy.[4] The latter is no longer questionable, and yet these products are still prescribed for use by hapless individuals. Aluminum antacids and phosphate binders are two medications that should be avoided by everyone if it is at all possible. Many will not appreciate that the buffer often included in many popular brand painkillers is an aluminum salt. Other well-known brands of painkillers include aluminum salts as lakes (commonly used term to describe aluminum compounds used to color products) to give tablets their distinctive color. These are products used regularly by millions of people completely unaware of their aluminum content. They represent significant exposure to aluminum by many, and choosing a type or brand of painkiller that does not include aluminum is highly recommended.

There are other insidious ways by which we are exposed to aluminum through regular use of medications. Fluoroquinolones are commonly prescribed antibiotics that, while not necessarily contaminated with aluminum (this is not yet known), are likely to bind aluminum in the gut and potentially increase its uptake into blood. I am reminded of recent press speculation reinforced by published medical research of a potential link between regular use of these antibiotics and poor mental health. Effects upon our mental health are certainly one outcome of chronic intoxication by aluminum. Of course, vaccines that include an aluminum adjuvant are significant contributors to the body burden of aluminum, especially in infants. I have written about this subject specifically elsewhere in this book, and I probably do not need to reiterate my opinion that I recommend avoiding vaccines that include an aluminum adjuvant whenever possible.

Insidious exposure to aluminum in medicine and clinical practice is a burgeoning issue. We have known for a long time that parenteral preparations, whether designed for use in premature babies or in nil-by-mouth

---

4 Christopher Exley, "What is the risk of aluminium as a neurotoxin?" *Expert Review of Neurotherapeutics* 14, no. 6 (April 30, 2014): 589-591, https://www.tandfonline.com/doi/full/10 .1586/14737175.2014.915745.

hospitalized adults, are contaminated with aluminum. Attempts by regulatory bodies to limit this contamination to 25 μg/L or ppb are largely symbolic and are not enforced. However, the recommendation of a limit for the aluminum content of parenteral solutions is evidence of an admission by governments that the perfusion of aluminum directly into the bloodstream is unacceptable. Therefore, it should be prevented wherever possible. What then of the latest revelations concerning the use of fluid-warming devices where contamination of transfused fluids—including whole blood—reached values in excess of 1000 μg/L?[5] That is fifty times the suggested limit for parenteral nutrition. Individuals, already severely ill, are being transfused with extraordinarily high levels of aluminum. It is impossible to know how long this practice has been in operation and how many people have died or suffered incomparable further illness because of this total lack of care and understanding. These fluid warmers remain in use today throughout the world. Lawyers are warming their hands in anticipation of the human fallout. While aluminum in warmed transfusions has only recently been brought to general attention, it has been known for many years that prosthetics are sources of systemic aluminum, from hip replacements to craniofacial prostheses, including myriad dental products. Usually there are prosthetics that are aluminum-free or at least have not been shown to leach aluminum once implanted. Again, given the opportunity, these should be the preferred options. Medications are unavoidable for many and form part of everyday living. Try to follow this rule: if medication is necessary, then choose one that does not include aluminum or does not predispose you to absorb more aluminum from your diet. The answers are not easily found, but in doing so you can help to lower your overall exposure to aluminum.

Cosmetics and Personal Care Products

Cosmetics, including personal care products, are an issue, as many include aluminum as an ingredient. Some, such as antiperspirants, are obvious, while others, including aluminum in sunscreen and sunblock, are less overt.[6] Often aluminum is present to aid in the manufacture or processing

5 Christopher Exley, "Aluminium release during fluid warming," *Anaesthesia* 74, no. 6 (June 2019): 819, https://onlinelibrary.wiley.com/doi/full/10.1111/anae.14673.

6 Scott Nicholson and Christopher Exley, "Aluminum: A potential pro-oxidant in sunscreens/ sunblocks?" *Free Radical Biology and Medicine* 43, no. 8 (Ocotber 15, 2007): 1216–1217, https://www.sciencedirect.com/science/article/abs/pii/S0891584907004911.

of the product, similarly to food, and while its inclusion should mean that it is listed as an ingredient, it may be as an E number or something equivalent. Cosmetics raise a number of additional concerns in that they are often applied liberally and regularly and sometimes to parts of the body where the potential for exposure is increased, such as in lipsticks.[7] Many years ago, I was asked by Procter & Gamble to assess the possible role of aluminum in antiperspirants in Alzheimer's disease. This was somewhat forward-thinking at the time for a pharmaceutical giant and, at times, an enjoyable consultation, since my P&G contact would meet me in London every two or three months for a working lunch at a fabulous Michelin-starred restaurant. Perhaps there is such a thing as a "free lunch"? Upon concluding the review of the evidence, my main piece of advice to them, subsequently published in the trends journal *Molecular Medicine Today*, was to discontinue the manufacture of antiperspirant aerosols.[8] It seemed inevitable to me that aerosols of aluminum-based antiperspirant would gain immediate access to the hippocampus of the brain via the olfactory route. Essentially, if you can smell your antiperspirant, then it is highly likely that not only the perfume element of the product has accessed your nose. Outside of the area of antiperspirants, there has been limited research on the contribution of cosmetics to human exposure to aluminum. It is no longer safe to assume that the skin is an impermeable barrier to any topical application. I am personally concerned about the nose and the lungs as routes of exposure to aluminum in any cosmetic applied as an aerosol.

As an interesting aside, I recall reading research that investigated airborne exposure to pollutants in individuals visiting active volcanoes. Stay with me: this is relevant. Participants provided urine samples both before and immediately after their visit, and the one major change recorded in all individuals was a significant increase in urinary excretion of aluminum. Only a brief exposure to volcano plumes resulted in immediate and significant excretion of aluminum in urine. The experiment demonstrates how quickly aluminum can enter the body simply by breathing polluted air.

---

7 Sa Liu, S. Katharine Hammond, and Ann Rojas-Cheatham, "Concentrations and Potential Health Risks of Metals in Lip Products," *Environmental Health Perspectives* 121, no. 6 (June 1, 2013) https://ehp.niehs.nih.gov/doi/10.1289/ehp.1205518.

8 Christopher Exley, "Does antiperspirant use increase the risk of aluminium-related disease, including Alzheimer's disease?" *Trends in Molecular Medicine* 4, no. 3 (March 1, 1998): 107–109, https://www.cell.com/trends/molecular-medicine/fulltext/S1357-4310(98)01209-X ?_returnURL=https%3A%2F%2Flinkinghub.elsevier.com%2Fretrieve%2Fpii%2FS1357 43109801209X%3Fshowall%3Dtrue.

The aluminum found within hours of first exposure probably represented absorption across the surfaces of the lungs; it is sobering to ask the fate of the aluminum that entered through the nose and subsequently the olfactory system. This aluminum may still be in the hippocampus of the brains of those naive participants in this experiment. Be wary of cosmetics as potential contributors to the body burden of aluminum and make informed and practical decisions about how to reduce exposure to aluminum through their regular use.

Social Habits

Recreational social habits can be significant contributors to the body burden of aluminum, particularly those involving inhalation through the nose or lungs. Remember that anything absorbed into the blood via the gut will have to pass through the liver before potentially accessing the rest of the body, including the brain. This means that there is an opportunity for some degree of detoxification. Aluminum in any form that is inhaled through the nose or the lung bypasses this first line of defense. Tobacco has long been associated with human disease and with lung cancer specifically. Sir Richard Doll in his seminal work[9] made it very clear that smoking tobacco is a significant environmental factor in the development of lung cancer, and indeed other respiratory diseases. However, Doll used epidemiology to demonstrate this link, and to this day, we still do not understand the mechanism whereby tobacco smoking increases the incidence of lung cancer. I have always been intrigued by "how" an agent causes a disease, and, with this in mind, I decided to investigate the aluminum content of tobacco.[10] We found that tobacco was aluminum-rich, not because the plant has any requirement for the metal, but, similar to tea and coffee, because many tobacco crops are grown on acidic soils allowing the adventitious accumulation of aluminum in the plant. By setting up a smoking machine in the laboratory, we also showed that aluminum in tobacco is biologically available in that it is trapped upon its passage through a surrogate lung fluid. These are sobering experiments to carry out. Smoke exiting the filter on a

9 "Sir Richard Doll," *The BMJ*, https://www.bmj.com/content/suppl/2005/07/28/331.7511 .295.DC1.

10 Christopher Exley, PhD, Amina Begum, BSc, Mark P. Woolley, MB, and Roger N. Bloor, PhD, "Aluminum in Tobacco and Cannabis and Smoking-Related Disease," *The American Journal of Medicine* 119, no. 3 (March 1, 2006): 276.E9-276.E11, https://www.amjmed.com /article/S0002-9343(05)00710-2/fulltext.

cigarette is thick and black, while it appears wispy and white exiting the surrogate lung fluid. Aluminum is part of the black retentate trapped by the surrogate lung fluid; it is little wonder that smoking contributes to lung disease. Smoking tobacco is a significant contributor to the body burden of aluminum, and I hypothesized that aluminum could be responsible for many smoking-related lung diseases.

Based on these interesting observations, I applied for a grant from one of the research foundations supported by the tobacco industry. The idea was to employ hydroponics to produce aluminum-free tobacco for toxicity testing in animal and human experiments. You will not be surprised to learn that this grant application was not successful. Tobacco is not only smoked; it is also mixed with a variety of different excipients and placed in the mouth, for example, immediately adjacent to the gums and is sometimes referred to as chewing tobacco. Nicotine is slowly released from the product and may be absorbed through the gums or the tongue, or it may be swallowed. Chewing tobacco is also associated with disease and specifically cancers of the mouth. We cannot know if the aluminum content of chewing tobacco plays a role in the diseases associated with its regular use. It is plausible, since, as is the case with smoking, nicotine is usually singled out as the toxin for particular attention.

The arrival on the market of electronic cigarettes might inadvertently herald an opportunity to test the toxicity of nicotine in smoking. The e-cigarette takes tobacco out of the equation and allows smoking of nicotine products in an inert vehicle. These products intrigued us, and we set about testing the aluminum content of e-liquids.[11] We also investigated whether or not a surrogate lung fluid would capture any aluminum released during vaping. The aluminum content of a wide range of e-liquids, including several rated as high in nicotine, was found to be almost negligible, at least in comparison to aluminum in tobacco. However, to our great surprise, when e-liquids were "vaped" in our laboratory smoking machine, the amount of aluminum collected by the surrogate lung fluid was much higher than we had seen previously for tobacco. We went on to find that the aluminum was not originating from the e-liquid, but from the heating element in the body of the e-cigarette used to vaporize the e-liquid. This immediately suggested that e-cigarettes were not going to be safe alternatives to smoking tobacco, and this has been borne out by a burgeoning body of research into their safety. One recent study likened lung damage following regular vaping to

---

11 Christopher Exley, "More to e-cigarettes than meets the eye?" *Tobacco Control* (September 27, 2017) https://tobaccocontrol.bmj.com/content/27/4/359.responses.

that which had been observed over many years of occupational exposure to metals. The experiment that remains to be carried out is one where e-liquids containing high amounts of nicotine (and preferably nothing else) are vaporized using a stainless steel (or at least aluminum-free) heating element. Long-term observation of individuals using this form of e-cigarette could go a long way toward establishing if aluminum (and/or nicotine) in tobacco is in fact responsible for some smoking-related diseases.

In related research, we also showed that street cannabis is aluminum-rich, as is pure tetrahydrocannabinol (THC), its active ingredient. In my opinion, this is sufficient to warn against the use of cannabis in human disease therapy, for example, multiple sclerosis. I make this warning with the proviso that the products tested were off the street and provided to us under license by the police. Cannabis grown hydroponically in the absence of aluminum should be aluminum-free and therefore could be used as a putative therapeutic agent.

Tobacco and cannabis are not the only recreational drugs that contribute toward the body burden of aluminum. Research elsewhere has shown that cocaine is heavily contaminated with aluminum, and this may be due to the presence of aluminum in the original plant tissue or, perhaps equally likely, the fact that aluminum is introduced into the product during its illegal processing. The latter is probably the case, since we did not find that street heroin, a related product, is contaminated with aluminum, at least not appreciably.[12] However, we did find very high levels of aluminum in the urine of heroin addicts. The answer to this particular conundrum probably comes down to the way in which heroin can be taken. In "chasing the dragon," the addict inhales heroin that has been vaporized off aluminum foil, which is a form of exposure to aluminum similar to vaporized e-liquids in e-cigarettes.

Recreational drugs, legal or otherwise, are significant contributors to the body burden of aluminum, and not using them will reduce your exposure to aluminum and, perhaps specifically, the brain's exposure to aluminum. It is almost certainly not a coincidence that early stages of neurodegeneration in Alzheimer's disease are consistently observed in the brain tissue of young heroin addicts dying of an overdose.

12 Christopher Exley, Usman Ahmed, Anthony Polwart, and Roger N. Bloor, "CLINICAL STUDY: Elevated urinary aluminium in current and past users of illicit heroin," *Addiction Biology* 12, no. 2 (June 2007): 197–199, https://onlinelibrary.wiley.com/doi/abs/10.1111/j.1369 -1600.2007.00055.x.

The Air We Breathe

The air that we breathe is largely unavoidable exposure to aluminum.[13] Aluminum is present in the air in myriad different forms, both natural, such as wind-blown dusts from across the globe, and unnatural, such as particulates from the incomplete combustion of fossil and other fuels. In our most polluted cities, we regularly breathe in particulate materials that are anything between a thousandth and a hundredth of a millimeter in size, often abbreviated as PMs with the notation PM10, meaning particulates of around 10 μm in size. Many PMs are aluminum-based or at least aluminum-rich. Everyday exposure to PMs is implicated in all manner of human disease, from respiratory disorders to neurological disease such as Alzheimer's disease. While we are a long way from attributing etiology to these correlative relationships, a contributory role for aluminum through exposure to PMs cannot and should not be discounted. The air that we breathe is also contaminated with aluminum residues from aircraft and rocket fuel. Aluminum is a powerful propellant, and without its inclusion in such fuels, it is unlikely that we would have made it out of Earth's atmosphere and onward and upward to the moon and beyond. Aerosols of aluminum salts are also proposed as tools for engineering climate. Applied as clouds in the upper atmosphere, they might act as coolants by reflecting and/or absorbing heat from the sun. There is a global body of activists believing that this activity, known as "geoengineering," is actually ongoing as opposed to being a suggestion for future consideration. Personally, I could think of few worse environmental practices than the wholesale contamination of the atmosphere with aluminum salts destined to fall to Earth. I have always taken my lead on environmental issues from independent peer-reviewed scientific literature, and, right now, this does not support the claims of the geoengineering activists. Indeed, we went as far as to use Keele University's designated meteorological station to collect dry and wet deposition over a period of twelve weeks from October to December 2015 and measure its content of aluminum. In spite of skies that were regularly decorated with what are called chemtrails, possibly contrails (flume from aircraft), and our usual amount of rainfall, we did not measure unusually high content of aluminum in either dry or wet deposition during this period. To investigate further the possibility that geoengineering using aerosols of

---

13 Christopher Exley, "Human exposure to aluminium," *Environmental Science: Processes & Impacts*, https://pubs.rsc.org/en/content/articlelanding/2013/EM/C3EM00374D#!divAbstract.

aluminum salts was being or had been practiced in the United Kingdom, we additionally obtained historical rainfall data for aluminum. This was from the Meteorological Office in the United Kingdom and covered a number of designated sites across the country. Again, there were no unusual or suspicious data to suggest that our atmosphere was or still is being actively contaminated with aluminum.

That is with one exceptional exception. The Summer 2012 readings for Porton Down in southern England were very high, at least ten times higher than the highest value recorded in our experiments at Keele. Whether these unusual data are evidence of an experiment in geoengineering in the United Kingdom, or perhaps over the Atlantic Ocean, is impossible to know. However, it is true that following the publication in 2009 of a report on geoengineering by the Royal Society of London, two of the United Kingdom's research councils, the Engineering and Physical Sciences Research Council (EPSRC) and the Natural Environment Research Council (NERC), convened a sandpit discussion on the subject. One outcome of this discussion was a project called SPICE (Stratospheric Particle Injection from Climate Engineer) to investigate the feasibility of using aerosols in climate change mitigation.[14] All information specific to this project has disappeared from the EPSRC website, and just one document, from 2011, remains on the NERC website. The scientists associated with SPICE were acutely aware of the controversial aspects of their work, and such may be behind the apparent closure of the project. Whether this project, and with it geoengineering, continues elsewhere in the United Kingdom (or around the world) is unknown. Until there is incontrovertible evidence to the contrary, I will continue to reserve judgement on its contribution to human exposure to aluminum. I very much hope that I am right!

Getting Aluminum Out of the Body

We can see how cutting out processed foods and drinks, over-the-counter medication, and overuse of prescribed medication, aluminum-containing cosmetics, and certain social habits associated with smoking and their equivalents will reduce your exposure to aluminum. However, equally important is what you can do to help your body to excrete aluminum.

Aluminum is naturally excreted from the body, though there is nothing "natural" about this. It is wholly adventitious, chaotic, even random and

14 "The SPICE Project," accessed September 30, 2020, http://www.spice.ac.uk/.

probably highly personalized. Aluminum accumulates in body tissues and fluids, and when these are shed or excreted, aluminum is lost from the body. The main vehicles carrying aluminum out of the body are feces, urine, sweat, skin, hair, nails, breast milk, semen, and other reproductive fluids. In theory at least, a faster turnover of all of these should help to facilitate increased excretion of aluminum. I say that excretion can be highly personalized to reflect the fact that we cannot be entirely sure, for any individual, which of the possible routes by which aluminum leaves the body is of greatest importance. The feces is clearly critical in the removal of aluminum that has not entered the systemic circulation, including some that is absorbed and then excreted via the liver and bile. It is largely assumed that urinary excretion is the main route of removal of aluminum from blood and tissues.

However, recent data on the aluminum content of sweat have highlighted the important role that perspiration plays in removing aluminum from the body. It may be equally important as urine and even more important in some individuals in certain circumstances. The role of sweating may be of particular significance in that the basal rate of perspiration in females is about half that of males, and this could suggest that females are predisposed to retain more aluminum in their bodies. The good news is that if sweating is an efficient way to remove aluminum from the body, then it is also a route by which the removal of aluminum could be increased, for example, through physical exercise or regular use of sauna. It is interesting to speculate that the higher incidence of Alzheimer's disease in women is related to their lower basal rate of sweating, while the known protective effects of both exercise and sauna against developing Alzheimer's disease could have something to do with increased sweating due to these activities.

Any activity or habit that has the potential to facilitate the removal of aluminum from the body is to be encouraged, and while some may be obvious, like those that increase perspiration volume, others may remain to be discovered and might include aspects of our diet. I have been asked so many times about the potential for certain foods, vitamins, and supplements to protect against the toxicity of aluminum. In truth, robust and reproducible scientific research in this field of study is sadly lacking. That is not to say that the scientific literature is not already awash with papers demonstrating the amelioration of aluminum toxicity in animal models. Myriad different treatments have been shown to be effective against the toxicity of aluminum, including many plant-based products, vitamins, small peptides, and amino acids. They are usually protective either because they prevent the uptake of aluminum into the body or because they address the symptoms of aluminum toxicity. The former is relatively easy to achieve in animal models of aluminum intoxication, as the beneficial agent is nearly always coadministered with the aluminum challenge, for example, in diet by gavage.[15] In humans in real life, we are exposed to aluminum continuously and by many different routes. Treatments that address the symptoms of aluminum intoxication are probably more practical than those attempting to reduce exposure to aluminum. For example, treatments that counter oxidative stress, though this approach may only be masking the issue of toxicity and may need to be undertaken on a regular basis for long periods. Therapies effective in animal models of aluminum intoxication have not been shown to increase the removal of aluminum from the body. This research includes a number of so-called chelation studies where molecules designed to bind aluminum are either injected directly into the bloodstream, inhaled as aerosols, or ingested with the view that they will facilitate the excretion of aluminum. While some of these animal studies have been effective in ameliorating some of the symptoms of aluminum intoxication, they have not been shown to achieve these effects by increased excretion of aluminum. One therapy has achieved this dual objective in animal models of intoxication by aluminum. It is the role played by drinking silicon-rich mineral waters in helping to protect the body against the toxicity of aluminum. The story behind this wonderful science is told elsewhere herein, and it is science that goes right back to the beginning of my aluminum story.

---

15 Caroline Silveira Martinez, Caroline D. C. Alterman, Gema Vera, Antonio Márquez, José-A Uranga, Franck Maciel Peçanha, Dalton Valentim Vassallo, Christopher Exley, Pâmela B. Mello-Carpes, Marta Miguel, and Giulia Alessandra Wiggers, "Egg White Hydrolysate as a functional food ingredient to prevent cognitive dysfunction in rats following long-term exposure to aluminum," *Scientific Reports* 9 (February 12, 2019) https://www.nature.com/articles/s41598-018-38226-7.

A Silicon-Rich Mineral Water a Day Keeps . . . Aluminum at Bay

Early Days

Some assaults on the senses imprint for life. One that remains with me is a smell that heralded salmon parr dead and dying from intoxication by aluminum. A parr is a juvenile salmon before it begins its journey from freshwater to the sea. I first encountered this fetid, though curiously sweet, aroma during undergraduate research into how aluminum interfered with the homing instinct of salmon. Well, death by aluminum proved to be the ultimate interference. Dead fish don't migrate and don't come home. Actually, as a brief aside, chronic intoxication by aluminum does interfere with homing instincts in salmon, and this may be one very good explanation of the reduced numbers of returning salmon in rivers and streams impacted by acid rain. I wrote about this in my first scientific publication, a chapter in a book on how acid rain was affecting salmon farming.[1]

This early research into aluminum toxicity in fish troubles me more now, nearly forty years later, than at the time. Observations of their death signatures, then recorded as disassociated data, feel strangely prescient when

---

1 Christopher Exley and Michael J. Phillips, "Acid Rain: Implications For The Farming of Salmonids," *Recent Advances in Aquaculture* (1988): 225-341, https://link.springer.com/chapter/10.1007/978-94-011-9743-4_4.

recalled today. Specifically so in the light of what we now know about aluminum's role in neurodevelopmental and neurodegenerative disease. Aluminum, at a concentration allowed in potable water under European Union law, kills a salmon parr within forty-eight hours of first exposure.[2] Only after eighteen hours do the fish show any obvious signs of distress. Their movements, within the confines of an experimental tank, begin to appear spasmodic, even frantic, as if searching for sanctuary from the poison. We learned only much later that fish actively avoid aluminum at concentrations less than one-twentieth of the aforementioned acutely toxic amount.[3] Quiet consolidation follows the escape response. Fish move toward the bottom and sides of the tank attempting to find solace away from wide-open spaces. They maintain this orientation, head pointed toward a corner of the tank, for as long as they have control over their actions. Before dying, their bodies stricken with involuntary muscle movements, they gasp at the surface of the tank, preferring air to their habitual water. The smell? Well this is evident within hours of death and may emanate from the copious quantities of mucus produced during the final thralls of life. Whatever its precise origin, it is a harbinger of death and one that now haunts my every day. However, it was not always like this. Early one morning on a spring day in 1988, I opened the airlock door of the temperature-controlled room that housed my experimental tanks, and, although I expected to be greeted by that smell, the air was, well, normal. This was my epiphany and my first indication of the seminal role played by silicon in protecting all living things from aluminum.[4]

Back to Today

As I sit contemplating and writing this part of my book, I am sipping on silicon-rich mineral water. This is something that I do each and every day, and why, you might ask, is that? As I have just recalled, the main finding of my PhD research, published in *Nature* in 1989, was that silicon protected

2 C. Exley, J. S. Chappell, and J. D. Birchall, "A mechanism for acute aluminium toxicity in fish," *Journal of Theoretical Biology* 151, no. 3 (August 7, 1991): 417–428, https://www.sciencedirect.com/science/article/abs/pii/S0022519305803893?via%3Dihub.

3 Christopher Exley, "Avoidance of aluminum by rainbow trout," *Environmental Toxicology and Chemistry* 19, no. 4 (April 2000): 933–939, https://setac.onlinelibrary.wiley.com/doi/abs/10.1002/etc.5620190421.

4 J. D. Birchall, C. Exley, J. S. Chappell, and M. J. Phillips, "Acute toxicity of aluminium to fish eliminated in silicon-rich acid waters," *Nature* 338 (March 9, 1989): 146–148, https://www.nature.com/articles/338146a0.

against the toxicity of aluminum in salmon. In the published paper, we added a "throwaway" line that I might paraphrase herein as "what is good for salmon should be good for us too." Research that followed my salmon paper suggested that silicon might protect against the toxicity of aluminum in humans by reducing its absorption across the gut. Intriguingly, this specific suggestion of reduced gastrointestinal absorption of aluminum by silicon remains somewhat equivocal even today. A subsequent observation that drinking beer increased the urinary excretion of aluminum raised some eyebrows, and we set about understanding the mechanism underlying this consistent effect. How might drinking beer help the body to remove aluminum? A suggestion that alcohol in some way might be involved was shown experimentally not to be the case. It was a follow-up observation that not all beers were equal in eliciting the increased content of aluminum in urine that gave us the clue that only beers rich in silicon affected urinary excretion of aluminum. Indeed, while the new research seemed to legitimize the beer-drinking habit that many of us espoused, thereafter it was quickly ascertained that it was drinking silicic acid, the soluble and biologically available form of silicon in beer, that facilitated the removal of aluminum from the body in urine.

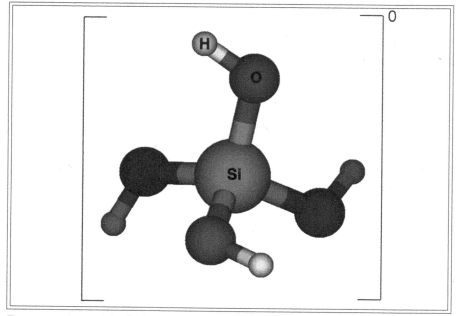

Figure 5. A model of silicic acid, the biologically available form of silicon. A central silicon atom is surrounded by four hydroxyl groups, giving an overall molecular charge of zero. *Courtesy of X. Lopez.* (See color version in insert.)

This finding was revelatory at the time, and the detailed underlying chemistry responsible continues at present to be largely unexplained. The best understanding of this effect that we have is that silicic acid follows water across the human gut into the blood, where, if its concentration is sufficiently high, it is bound by aluminum hydroxide. Note, we are not talking about silicic acid being bound by biologically reactive aluminum, $Al^{3+}_{(aq)}$, but by the insoluble product of its hydrolysis $[Al(OH)_3]_n$ where n must be greater than or equal to 2. The presence of insoluble aluminum hydroxide in blood is actually equivocal, and its existence in blood has only been proven in a computational model, though, if I may say so, an exceptional computational model from my group.[5] What we have proven, in what already feels like a lifetime of science, is that when silicic acid is bound by aluminum hydroxide, it forms what we have called hydroxyaluminosilicates. These small amorphous solids, though ultimately prone to aggregation, should remain small enough for long enough to be filtered from the blood by the kidney. While I am personally convinced that this is the mechanism whereby silicic acid facilitates the removal of aluminum from the body in urine, it is only a hypothesis and remains to be proven. The science underlying the formation of hydroxyaluminosilicates in water, as opposed to the more complex medium of blood, has, with the help of an exceptional scientist and my good friend, Xabier Lopez from the University of San Sebastian, been proven.[6] When funding permits, I am sure we will extend this seminal research to what is happening in the human bloodstream and, thereafter, urine.

To truly appreciate what is being touted here, the reader needs to understand that the chemistry of silicic acid in the natural environment is extremely limited; one might say that its interaction with aluminum is its only chemistry of true biological significance. Silicic acid does react with itself when its solubility is exceeded, and this is the basis for a process called silicification, an important mechanism in plants and some simple animals.[7]

---

5 James Beardmore and Christopher Exley, "Towards a model of non-equilibrium binding of metal ions in biological systems," *Journal of Inorganic Biochemistry* 103, no. 2 (February 2009): 205–209, https://www.sciencedirect.com/science/article/pii/S0162013408002468?via%3Dihub.

6 James Beardmore, Xabier Lopez, Jon I. Mujika, and Christopher Exley, "What is the mechanism of formation of hydroxyaluminosilicates?" *Scientific Reports* 6 (August 1, 2016) https://www.nature.com/articles/srep30913.

7 Christopher Exley, "Silicon in Life: Whither Biological Silicification?" *Biosilica in Evolution, Morphogenesis, and Nanobiotechnology* 47 (2009): 173–184, https://link.springer.com/chapter/10.1007/978-3-540-88552-8_7.

The next obvious step following the identification of silicic acid as the "magical" ingredient was to identify a product, preferably nonalcoholic, that would be a good source of it. Since silicic acid is the most natural of natural products—after all, it derives from the rainfall-fueled dissolution of the Earth's crust—a natural mineral water should be an obvious choice. However, a trip to the local supermarket revealed that there were no mineral waters of UK origin that contained a high level of silicic acid. I should not have been surprised by this, since the United Kingdom is a heavily eroded (geologically old) land mass from which the majority of the crustal silicic acid has already been leached over preceding millions of years. When the Earth's crust is newly formed, it is silicon-rich, and its incongruent dissolution by incipient rainfall leads to the leaching of high amounts of silicic acid. The latter forms soil solutions, lakes, and rivers and may even be collected deeper down in the Earth in ground waters and artesian wells. Of course, over time the silicic acid in all of these freshwater reservoirs empties into the oceans and, with increasing dissolution of parent rocks, is replaced at a slower and slower rate leading to lower overall levels of silicic acid in our natural freshwaters.[8]

To find a natural water rich in silicic acid, we have to look further afield. One that I found in my local supermarket was called Volvic and originated from a region in France with relatively recent geology, including volcanic activity (hence the name of the water). The silicon content of Volvic is approximately 30 mg/L or ppm, expressed as silica (a quirk of the water industry: there is not, or at least should not be, any silica in these natural waters), which is about 14 mg/L as silicic acid. Having identified what I hoped would be a suitable water, I was quick to cut to the chase and I contacted my colleague Peter Crome in Neurology at Keele to suggest a small clinical trial involving individuals with Alzheimer's disease. Professor Crome is one of those rare clinical scientists who is not afraid to step on the toes of the pharmaceutical industry if there is an opportunity to do good, sound science. He was the lead author on the 2000 study that demonstrated unequivocally, once and for all, that Aricept (donepezil), a drug that continues to make its manufacturer millions of pounds, has no benefit in treating Alzheimer's disease.

In the spirit of many great advances in medicine, I began by experimenting upon myself, and, as a willing "healthy volunteer," I quickly

---

8 Christopher Exley, Gea Guerriero, and Xabier Lopez, "Silicic acid: The omniscient molecule," *Science of The Total Environment* 665 (May 15, 2019): 432–437, https://www .sciencedirect.com/science/article/abs/pii/S0048969719306862?via%3Dihub.

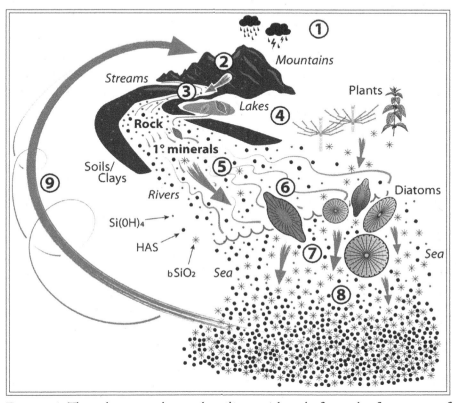

Figure 6. The schematic shows the silicic acid cycle from the formation of silicic acid through to its eventual deposition in sediments of rivers, lakes, and seas. Please see the full paper for a complete explanation of numbers and abbreviations.** (See color version in insert.)

** Ibid.

demonstrated the removal of aluminum from my body through simply drinking 1.5L of Volvic. We then wanted to know whether the same would be achieved in individuals with Alzheimer's disease. It then followed that the most difficult aspect of the proposed clinical trial was in obtaining ethical approval for asking individuals with a diagnosis of Alzheimer's disease to drink Volvic. Perhaps it was the simplicity of what we were suggesting that confused the ethical committee. While we waited for final approval from our National Research Ethics Committee (NREC), I wrote several letters and emails to individuals within the hierarchy at Volvic to inform them of our plans and to ascertain if they would be interested in supporting the research in some way. No one replied to any of these communications. We went ahead with the trial as planned and stripped the shelves of the local supermarket of Volvic.

The clinical trial was a success.[9] As a proof of concept, it showed that regular drinking of a silicon-rich mineral water, Volvic, over just five consecutive days facilitated the urinary excretion of aluminum in individuals with a diagnosis of Alzheimer's disease. The research was published in the *Journal of Alzheimer's Disease*, and almost immediately following I received a telephone call and email from someone from Volvic. Of course, they denied receiving any previous correspondence from me on this matter but they were, they said, intrigued by the research, and I was invited to Danone's (Volvic's parent company) Paris headquarters to discuss future possibilities. This proved to be a mutually agreeable first meeting, with the eventual outcome of several months of further discussion being a signed contract between Danone and Keele University. Volvic would provide funding (£30,000) and resources to partially support a PhD and to enable us to carry out a follow-up clinical trial over a longer period of time. We also planned to perform additional studies involving healthy volunteers. Only six months into the signed contract, I received a conference telephone call from my contact at Volvic informing me that they were pulling out of the project. No clear reason for breaking the contract was offered by Volvic.

However, my understanding of the French language, having lived in Belgium for five years, allowed me to overhear voices in the background of the conference call. These voices were making it clear to my contact that he

9 Christopher Exley et al., "Non-invasive therapy to reduce the body burden of aluminium in Alzheimer's disease," *Journal of Alzheimer's Disease* 10, no. 1 (2006): 17–24, https://content.iospress.com/articles/journal-of-alzheimers-disease/jad00618?resultNumber=18&totalResults=80&start=10&q=Exley+2006&resultsPageSize=10&rows=10.

should not give me a specific reason behind them pulling out of the contract. Later, the official reason given was that the proposed research with Volvic mineral water clashed with Danone's other research on Alzheimer's disease. My contact finished our conversation by stating that I should not "advertise" any of the previous involvement with Danone at any time in the future. Anyone reading this account and remaining incredulous at the sudden "cloak-and-dagger" response from Volvic needs to appreciate that Danone, a global nutrition company, makes extensive use of aluminum both in products and in packaging. They presumably made the decision that they could not risk any suggestion that they are supporting research that clearly identifies aluminum as toxic in humans. It would seem that the existence of a research contract investigating the health effects of aluminum did not go over well once it had been picked up within the higher echelons of the company. I do like to imagine their panic when this information was presented at a regular board meeting. It seems that those at Volvic, a small part of Danone, got their proverbial bottoms smacked once the news of the contract with Keele went upstairs in Danone.

However, the PhD project continued, and we found a new supplier (Spritzer from Malaysia)[10] for the thousands of liters of mineral water needed for the proposed new Alzheimer's disease clinical trial. The new trial involved individuals diagnosed with Alzheimer's disease and their caregiver or spouse drinking up to 1.5L of Spritzer every day for twelve weeks. The Spritzer mineral water arrived by ship, and we needed a number of healthy volunteers to help to carry many boxes of water to the large room where it was stored prior to being used in the trial. Even a relatively small clinical trial over just twelve weeks can be a logistical challenge if nothing else. The clinical trial was a tremendous success both in demonstrating that regular drinking of Spritzer, a silicon-rich mineral water, lowered the body burden of aluminum in individuals with Alzheimer's disease, but also, in three of the fifteen individuals, the fall in body burden of aluminum was paralleled by clinically relevant improvements in their cognitive function.

Let me reiterate this remarkable finding. Just twelve weeks of drinking up to 1.5L/day of Spritzer resulted in three of the fifteen participants with Alzheimer's disease having significantly improved cognitive abilities. Cognitive function in the remaining twelve participants remained unaltered after the twelve weeks of the trial. I challenge anyone reading this now to inform me about any trial of any drug for Alzheimer's disease where 20

---

10 Spritzer home page, accessed September 30, 2020, https://corporate.spritzer.com.my/.

percent of the participants showed clinically significant improvements in cognitive function by the end of the trial. This potentially landmark study was also published in the *Journal of Alzheimer's Disease*,[11] and at the time I hoped that it would prove to be the catalyst required to find the funding needed for a once and for all clinical trial testing the aluminum hypothesis of Alzheimer's disease. Of course, I am still waiting for this clinical trial. Perhaps one day.

However, the study was a catalyst for a crowdfunding initiative organized by the Washington, DC-based charity, Children's Medical Safety Research Institute (CMSRI),[12] to raise the money required to do a once-in-a-lifetime clinical trial to test the efficacy of silicon-rich mineral water as a therapy in Alzheimer's disease.[13] The platform chosen to host this initiative, Future Science, was new and inexperienced, and the funding goal of raising £500,000 was, in hindsight, almost certainly unrealistic for the early days of crowdfunding of life science projects. However, this ultimately unsuccessful initiative did have a silver lining of sorts. It generated significant press interest, and a man named Derek Garratt contacted me having heard an interview I gave at BBC Radio Stoke. He was fascinated by our research and had a personal interest in Malaysia, the origin of the Spritzer mineral water used in our previous clinical trial. Just a few days after this, I was contacted this time by his brother, Rex Garratt, who informed me that he was planning to approach Spritzer with an offer to set up an import agreement with them to bring Spritzer mineral water to the United Kingdom. The rest, as the saying goes, is history, and Spritzer mineral water is now available as the brand Acilis in the United Kingdom, Europe, and South Africa, solely due to the efforts of Rex Garratt.

This character deserves an aside, a special mention. Rex was a retired journalist when he contacted me. While he possessed some entrepreneurial flair, his motivation for setting up his company SilicaWaters[14] to sell Acilis (silica backward) was completely selfless. Over numerous discussions with me, he was aware that we were unable to obtain funding to continue our

---

11 Samantha Davenward et al., "Silicon-Rich Mineral Water as a Non-Invasive Test of the 'Aluminum Hypothesis' in Alzheimer's Disease," *Journal of Alzheimer's Disease* 33, no. 2 (2013): 423–430, https://content.iospress.com/articles/journal-of-alzheimers-disease/jad121231.

12 The Children's Medical Safety Research Institute (CMSRI) home page, accessed September 30, 2020, https://www.cmsri.org/.

13 "Aluminium and Alzheimer's disease: Time to test the link," accessed September 30, 2020, https://www.youtube.com/watch?v=jnsqeAi-v7M.

14 Silica Waters home page, accessed September 30, 2020, https://www.silicawaters.com/.

research into the potential health benefits of silicon-rich mineral waters such as Acilis. He set up the company SilicaWaters with the overall objective of making it successful so that any profits accrued by the company would be offered to Keele University to support our research on silicon and aluminum. It was truly business as a social enterprise. Rex Garratt is magnanimity personified, and he is a personal hero of mine and, I am proud to say, a friend.

Keele University, on the other hand, refused to allow me to accept this generous offer. As you will read later in the book, Keele is not averse to accepting millions of pounds from a local online betting company but felt that it would be compromised by accepting a much, much smaller amount of support from a local company selling a mineral water. Nevertheless, enthusiasm undiminished, Rex uses any small profits made by SilicaWaters to provide interested groups with Acilis mineral water free of charge. The company is currently run as an accredited social enterprise, and I fully endorse its aims and objectives.

There remain many unknowns concerning the role played by silicon-rich mineral waters in facilitating the removal of aluminum from the body. We hope that funding will eventually become available to test further hypotheses in this field. However, in the meantime, I consider silicon-rich mineral waters as a philosophy for living in the Aluminum Age as opposed to a classical "detox" therapy for aluminum.[15] This is why I drink one bottle every day: it is preventative as well as restorative. To provide continuous protection against the possibility of aluminum toxicity, try to drink about 1L/day of any mineral water where the content of silicon is above 30 mg/L (or ppm) when labeled (erroneously) as silica or 14 mg/L when labeled as silicic acid or just silicon. You can drink this in several small volumes throughout the day or in just two or three larger volumes when it is convenient. Make this a habit, just as drinking water on a daily basis should be for healthy living.

Currently there are no effective alternatives to natural silicon-rich mineral waters. See the Silicon Fact Sheet included in this chapter. There are myriad and burgeoning so-called silicon and silica supplements available through health stores and elsewhere, many of which are advertised by their suppliers to be effective in removing aluminum from the body. Some selling such products even falsely cite my research in support of this. These claims are groundless, and they are not supported by independent, peer-reviewed

---

15 "MetDetox: Silicic Acid: Nature's 'detox' for aluminium," accessed September 30, 2020, https://www.youtube.com/watch?v=1GB_MNIdg_k&t=880s.

published science. However, this does not mean that some of these supplements might not have health benefits, only that any such benefits are not accrued through the facilitated removal of aluminum from the body. When a health claim is made for a product, ask the company selling it to provide independently reviewed scientific proof, and preferably peer-reviewed publications, to support their claims. In particular, ask for studies that have shown that the product is actually safe for human consumption. Specifically relating to safety, I want to take this opportunity to warn you against suggestions on the Internet that you can make your own silicon-rich mineral water. You cannot. Preparation of something equivalent to a silicon-rich mineral water requires sophisticated laboratory equipment. In my laboratory we prepare water that is high in dissolved silicon—silicic acid—for research purposes. However, under no circumstances would I advocate drinking this water. Unless water is made or bottled under conditions that have been proven to be biologically safe, you cannot produce a drinking water that is safe for human consumption. Even in a sophisticated laboratory such as my own. Do not believe what you read and watch on the Internet: you cannot make a silicon-rich mineral water. Only Nature can do this.

The safety and efficacy of natural silicon-rich mineral waters are based upon many years of peer-reviewed published science. For example, following the clinical trial with individuals with a diagnosis of Alzheimer's disease, we did secure funding for a small clinical trial testing the efficacy of silicon-rich mineral water to lower the body burden of aluminum in individuals with multiple sclerosis. You can read the background to this trial elsewhere in this book, but the trial was successful in getting aluminum out of the body of people suffering with multiple sclerosis.[16]

I have been heard to say on more than one occasion that "myriad anecdotes doth not a clinical trial make," and while this is true, it has not prevented me from recommending silicon-rich mineral waters to anyone contacting me with a personal suspicion that they are suffering from some form of aluminum-related condition. I will continue to make such recommendations both because I believe in the preventative nature of silicon-rich mineral waters and because of the positive reports of their benefits that I have received in relation to Alzheimer's disease, multiple sclerosis, autism,

16 Krista Jones, Caroline Linhart, Clive Hawkins, and Christopher Exley, "Urinary Excretion of Aluminium and Silicon in Secondary Progressive Multiple Sclerosis," *EBioMedicine* 26 (December 1, 2017): 60–67, https://www.thelancet.com/journals/ebiom/article/PIIS2352 -3964(17)30428-0/fulltext.

epilepsy, and vaccine injury. I write this as I take a further sip from my glass of Acilis and wish you good health.

Human Exposure to Aluminium
Fact Sheet

Why Only Silicon-Rich Mineral Waters (and not silicon/silica supplements) Will Protect You from Aluminium

Silicic acid is the form of silicon which is found in silicon-rich mineral waters and is the only form of silicon in the diet which can pass rapidly from the gut to the bloodstream to help to remove aluminium from the body in the urine.

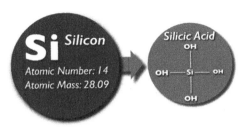

Si Silicon
Atomic Number: 14
Atomic Mass: 28.09

Silicic Acid

$$OH - Si - OH$$

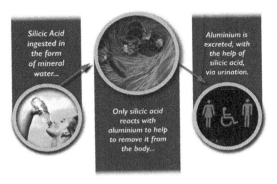

Silicic Acid ingested in the form of mineral water...

Only silicic acid reacts with aluminium to help to remove it from the body...

Aluminium is excreted, with the help of silicic acid, via urination.

When you drink a silicon-rich mineral water the silicic acid in the water passes immediately from your gut and into your blood producing a temporary rapid increase in the silicic acid in your blood. It is this temporary high concentration of silicic acid in the blood which reacts with aluminium in the blood and helps the aluminium to be removed from the body in the urine.

For more information, visit cmsri.org

The Only Biologically Available Form of Silicon is <u>Silicic Acid</u>
(neutral monomer, pka ~ 9.6, Ksp ~ 2 mmol/L)

A high level of silicic acid in the blood is essential to ensure that the product it makes with aluminium remains stable for long enough for it to be filtered by the kidney.

This is why only silicon-rich mineral waters, where the silicon content is above 30 mg/L or ppm when stated as 'silica'* or 14 mg/L or ppm when stated as 'silicon' or 'silicic acid' (sometimes written as OSA, orthosilicic acid), will help to remove aluminium from the body.

*Some confusion comes from the fact that 'historically' silicon in natural waters has been measured as 'silica' and the term silica is often seen on a mineral water bottle

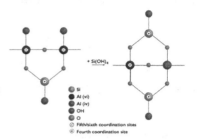

"We have investigated and tested every so-called silicon/silica supplement which is available to buy and not one of them can provide a high and immediate level of silicic acid for absorption across the gut and into the blood."

Professor Christopher Exley PhD, FRSB

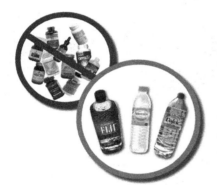

Exley C, Korchazhkina O, Job D, Strekopytov S, Polwart A & Crome P (2006) Non-invasive therapy to reduce the body burden of aluminium in Alzheimer's disease. Journal of Alzheimer's Disease 10, 17-24.
Davenward S, Bentham P, Wright J, Crome P, Job, D, Polwart A and Exley C (2013) Silicon-rich mineral water as a non-invasive test of the 'aluminium hypothesis' in Alzheimer's disease. Journal of Alzheimer's Disease 33, 423-430.
Beardmore J, Lopez X, Mujika JI and Exley C (2016) What is the mechanism of formation of hydroxyaluminosilicates? Scientific Reports 6:30913.
Jones K, Linhart C, Hawkins C, Exley C (2017) Urinary excretion of aluminium and silicon in secondary progressive multiple sclerosis. EBioMedicine
(http://www.ebiomedicine.com/article/S2352-3964(17)30428-0/fulltext)

For more information, visit cmsri.org

CHAPTER 10

Pregnancy and Why Infant Exposure to Aluminum Is a Special Case

How is human exposure to aluminum influencing everyday living, health, and well-being? What is its impact upon something as fundamental as reproductive success? From the quality of eggs and sperm, to fertilization, implantation, development of the fetus, successful birth, and, finally, a healthy infant, I am sure that it is already clear to everyone reading this book that the Aluminum Age guarantees our exposure to aluminum, and commensurately its biological reactivity ensures that all biochemical systems, all of our tissues and organs, are potential targets of aluminum's toxicity. Since I have your attention, you will already appreciate the need to reduce your personal exposure to aluminum. However, are there also additional steps that you can take to improve your fecundity in the Aluminum Age?

Reliable and robust scientific research relating to how aluminum affects human reproduction remains scarce. However, there are sufficient indications across scientific literature to suggest that its effects are more widespread than currently acknowledged.[1] A limited but significant body of

---

1 Halina B. Röllin, Kalavati Channa, Bukola Olutola, Claudina Nogueira, and Jon Ø. Odland, "In Utero Exposure to Aluminium and Other Neurotoxic Elements in Urban Coastal South African Women at Delivery: An Emerging Concern," *International Journal of Environmental Research and Public Health* 17, no. 5 (March 6, 2020): 1724, https://www.mdpi.com/1660-4601/17/5/1724.

research documents observations such as high concentrations of aluminum in human placental tissue[2] and even in the tissues of miscarried fetuses. The developing baby shares the mother's body burden of aluminum. There is published science that unequivocally equates the aluminum content of blood serum in pregnancy with congenital defects in the fetus.[3] There are similar data for aluminum in amniotic fluid, the fluid that bathes the fetus, and concomitant growth and health of the fetus and neonate. While these studies are relatively rare, they tell a consistent and worrying story of exposure to aluminum. It is, perhaps, not a surprise to find that biologically reactive aluminum exerts its affects throughout the human life cycle.

Research in my laboratory has shown that seminal fluid, semen, is a sink for aluminum in men, meaning its concentration of aluminum far exceeds, for example, that found in blood.[4] We found a statistically significant influence of aluminum in lowering sperm count. The higher the concentration of aluminum in semen, the lower the number of sperm in semen. Could human exposure to aluminum be a contributing factor in the now-well-documented lower sperm count in men in the developed world? Perhaps equally worrying is our observation using aluminum-specific fluorescence microscopy that some of the aluminum in semen is concentrated in the nuclei of sperm. We did not find any direct relationship between the aluminum content of semen and the motility and immediate viability of sperm, which suggests that aluminum-loaded sperm are in competition with normal, "aluminum-free" sperm to fertilize available eggs. Since the nucleus of the sperm is the critical "bit" passed on in fertilization, then this would imply that aluminum is also passed to the egg. While it is impossible to know, I would have to assume that aluminum passed on from sperm nucleus to egg

2 Pamela C. Kruger, Lawrence M. Schell, Alice D. Starke, and Patrick J. Parsons, "A study of the distribution of aluminium in human placental tissues based on alkaline solubilization with determination by electrothermal atomic absorption spectrometry," *Metallomics* 9, no. 2 (August 17, 2010): 621–627, https://pubs.rsc.org/en/content/articlelanding/2010/MT/c0mt00010h#!divAbstract.

3 Jacopo Troisi, Luigi Giugliano, Laura Sarno, Annamaria Landolfi, Sean Richards, Steven Symes, Angelo Colucci, Giuseppe Maruotti, David Adair, Marco Guida, Pasquale Martinelli, and Maurizio Guida, "Serum metallome in pregnant women and the relationship with congenital malformations of the central nervous system: a case-control study," *BMC Pregnancy and Childbirth* 19 (December 5, 2019) https://bmcpregnancychildbirth.biomedcentral.com/articles/10.1186/s12884-019-2636-5#Abs1.

4 J. P. Klein, M. Mold, L. Mery, M. Cottier, and C. Exley, "Aluminum content of human semen: Implications for semen quality," *Reproductive Toxicology* 50 (December 2014): 43–48, https://www.sciencedirect.com/science/article/abs/pii/S0890623814002548?via%3Dihub.

in the process of fertilization could not be an entirely benign interaction. It must have some influence; whether its affect is to prevent successful fertilization, subsequent division of the egg, the egg's implantation in the uterus, or the development of the fetus is, as yet, unknown in humans.

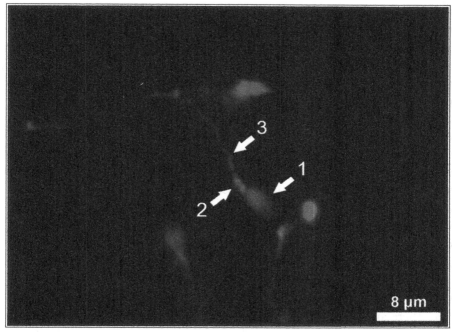

Figure 7. Aluminum-specific fluorescence microscopy shows the presence of aluminium as orange fluorescence in the head (1), midpiece (2), and tail of individual human sperm. Please see the full paper for further information.** (See color version in insert.)

However, there are myriad studies of aluminum intoxication in animals demonstrating effects upon all aspects of the reproductive cycle. It would seem inconceivable that similar effects are not already happening in humans. For example, dialysis encephalopathy in which exposure to aluminum—in dialysate as well as phosphate-controlling drugs—is heavily implicated could be considered as an unfortunate human model of intoxication by aluminum. Postmortem analyses of affected individuals reveal the presence of aluminum in both testes and ovaries. It would be naive to assume that such

** J. P. Klein, M. Mold, L. Mery, M. Cottier, and C. Exley, "Aluminum content of human semen: Implications for semen quality," *Reproductive Toxicology* 50 (December 2014): 43–48, https://www.sciencedirect.com/science/article/abs/pii/S0890623814002548?via%3Dihub.

deposits are only benign. Other aluminum-based medications implicated in reproductive health include aluminum adjuvants in vaccines. Numerous studies have identified vaccines that include an aluminum adjuvant as being involved in primary ovarian insufficiency and other issues of reproductive health.[5] The potential telltale signs of aluminum's involvement in human fecundity are out there, especially so in the advanced stages of the human experiment of the developed world (did we previously call it the first world?) where the decline in reproductive success is increasingly evident.

There is a significant market for supplements targeting reproductive success aimed at both men and women. These can be in tablet, capsule, or liquid form and usually entail daily consumption over extended periods. However, some multivitamin and mineral complexes intended to be taken both to increase the chance of becoming pregnant and, thereafter, for the subsequent health of the fetus up until birth are heavily contaminated with aluminum. Following the recommended guidelines on taking these supplements would result in the ingestion of ten to twenty milligrams of aluminum in this critical period. This represents a significant addition to an individual's daily consumption of aluminum beyond their normal everyday exposure. We have only been able to measure the aluminum content of a small fraction of these supplements, and it is advisable to read contents lists as closely as possible; if doubt still exists then in this connected world, send the manufacturer an email asking about the aluminum content of a product. There are changes that we can make to improve our chance of reproductive success in the Aluminum Age. However, what about the health of neonates and infants?

Birth releases the infant from the mother's body burden of aluminum. Well, at least directly, since an infant's only immediate source of nutrition is either breast milk, hence back to the mother's exposure to aluminum, or infant formula. I gave a lecture at AutismOne in Chicago in 2015 where I made the case, seriously if tongue in cheek, that an infant is an ideal model organism for human studies on intoxication by aluminum.[6] Ideal because infants above all other independent human forms are predisposed to take up aluminum into the body and retain it in the tissues. Several critical

5 Gayle DeLong, "Letters to the editor; Response to: a possible spurious correlation between human papillomavirus vaccination introduction and birth rate change in the United States," *Human Vaccines & Immunotherapeutics* 15, no. 10 (June 18, 2019): 2503–2504, https://www.tandfonline.com/doi/full/10.1080/21645515.2019.1622977.

6 "Christopher Exley, PhD, "Human Exposure to Aluminium," accessed September 30, 2020, http://www.autismone.org/content/christopher-exley-phd-human-exposure-aluminium.

physiological factors contribute toward such a predisposition. The infant gut is premature in that it is still developing, and in its nascent form, it is more permeable to aluminum in the diet. Upon aluminum entering the blood, the infant kidney is also far from being functionally complete, and so its capacity to remove aluminum from the blood is lower. Subsequently, when higher concentrations of aluminum circulating in the blood come into contact with a significantly underdeveloped blood-brain-barrier, the inevitable consequence is higher uptake of aluminum into brain tissue. Put each of these susceptibility factors together with the knowledge that an infant's capacity to excrete aluminum in urine and sweat is also not fully developed, and you have the ideal (as a model of aluminum intoxication) or nightmare (as a model of infant health) scenario of increased uptake concomitant with reduced excretion of aluminum.

Your child begins its independent life deriving its nourishment from its mother's breast, if it is lucky. Breast milk is a source of aluminum, and how much aluminum is in breast milk will depend upon a mother's exposure to aluminum during lactation, as well as simply a mother's overall body burden of aluminum. The good news is that in general the aluminum content of breast milk is low, at least in comparison to the only other alternative, infant formula. For a wide variety of reasons, from medical to societal, not all mothers are able to or choose to breast-feed their infant. A sad reality is that in the developed world, breastfeeding is a significant minority, and the majority of parents are choosing to use infant formulas within days of giving birth. All infant formulas tested in our laboratory are contaminated with aluminum, and many are *heavily* contaminated with aluminum.[7] For example, we are inadvertently feeding our infants milk formula that contains up to ten times the aluminum concentration allowed in drinking water under EU legislation. (As an aside and before you start to think that there is health-based legislation for aluminum: The EU maximum for the aluminum content of drinking water, 0.200 mg/L, is not a health-based limit; it is solely based upon the residual concentration, following water treatment with aluminum salts, which leaves the water with a crystal-clear appearance.)

7 Shelle-Ann M Burrell and Christopher Exley, "There is (still) too much aluminium in infant formulas," *BMC Pediatrics* 10 (August 31, 2010) https://bmcpediatr.biomedcentral.com/articles/10.1186/1471-2431-10-63.

All infant formulas contain too much aluminum;[8] soya-based formulas are some of the worst, while the highest levels of contamination are reserved for many of the formulas available on prescription for premature infants, term infants struggling to gain weight, and term infants with significant allergies and intolerances.[9] If you were designing a nutritional scandal, you simply could not come up with a worse scenario than that which already describes infant formula feeding. What would be the most effective way to load up newborn infants with a known neurotoxin? Of course, formula feeding is the perfect, even ideal, answer. This is an outrage, and one can only hope that this laissez-faire attitude toward infant health and nutrition will come home to roost upon manufacturers in the not-too-distant future. They will not be in a position to plead ignorance or even shift the responsibility onto someone else. Infant formula manufacturers have known about the issue of product contamination by aluminum for decades and have chosen to ignore a problem that they are *allowed* to ignore due to inaction by organizations such as the EFSA and FDA, which are charged with the responsibility of protecting the public from poisons in the food they eat.

There is much debate as to the origin of the contaminating aluminum. Manufacturers claim that they "no longer" add aluminum to their products. Note that they certainly used to, in the same way that all manufacturers of powdered nutritional products added aluminum salts to prevent their product from clumping. For example, aluminum was added to powdered milk products, such as whiteners, to make them free-flowing. Aluminum coats the milk powder, preventing it from forming aggregates either during its processing or in its packaging. Today, manufacturers of such products claim that these practices have been discontinued. One might question why they made this decision and who is monitoring if they are compliant. If we had not decided over ten years ago to look again at the aluminum content of infant formulas, then their widespread contamination may not be so widely known as it is today. So, if the manufacturers are no longer adding aluminum to their products, then why are their infant formulas so heavily contaminated? A possible explanation is that infant formula manufacturers buy

---

8 Nancy Chuchu, Bhavini Patel, Blaise Sebastian, and Christopher Exley, "The aluminium content of infant formulas remains too high," *BMC Pediatrics* 13 (October 8, 2013) https://bmcpediatr.biomedcentral.com/articles/10.1186/1471-2431-13-162.

9 James Redgrove, Isabel Rodriguez, Subramanian Mahadevan-Bava, and Christopher Exley, "Prescription Infant Formulas Are Contaminated with Aluminium," *International Journal of Environmental Research and Public* 16, no. 5 (March 12, 2019): 899, https://www.mdpi.com/1660-4601/16/5/899.

in their ingredients and only "assemble" the final products that they sell as formulas. It is most likely that aluminum is, added or otherwise, in the basic ingredients, including such integral constituents as whey protein hydrolysates. Indeed, we recently measured the aluminum content of whey protein hydrolysates for Arla, a major manufacturer, and found them to be heavily contaminated with aluminum. This is just one of many ingredients that make up infant formulas. My intuition tells me that whey protein hydrolysates are not the only ingredient that will be contaminated by aluminum. I am guessing, but I am also confident, that formula manufacturers do not ask their suppliers if their products are contaminated with aluminum. They cannot pass the buck of responsibility so easily.

To protect the product from oxidation and give enhanced shelf life, infant formulas are nearly always supplied in aluminum-based packaging. While packaging is a source of contamination of product, either powder or ready-to-drink, it is unlikely to be the major source. For example, we have found one or two prescription infant formulas where contamination by aluminum was low and almost, by the very low standards of the industry in general, acceptable. These products were contained within aluminum-based packaging, but, perhaps critically, their cost was almost ten times that of an off-the-shelf product, demonstrating that where ingredients are of high quality and therefore purity, the level of contamination by aluminum is concomitantly much lower. This, if nothing else, demonstrates that cost and greed underlie the contamination of infant formulas by aluminum. Profit margin for manufacturers is considered more important than the immediate and long-term health of infants. There is a significant body of historical evidence within the scientific literature linking aluminum in infant formula to infant health. Recent literature adds to these warnings and asks for action in reducing infants' exposure to aluminum.[10] However, there is no evidence that any steps are being taken either by manufacturers or regulatory agencies to protect infants from the toxicity of aluminum in infant formulas. While research has demonstrated immediate toxicity in infants by aluminum, we have to ask about latent toxicity. Infant formulas are a major contributor to the body burden of aluminum in infants, and it is inevitable that some

---

10 Daniela Fanni, Rossano Ambu, Clara Gerosa, Sonia Nemolato, Nicoletta Iacovidou, Peter Van Eyken, Vassilios Fanos, Marco Zaffanello, and Gavino Faa, "Aluminum exposure and toxicity in neonates: a practical guide to halt aluminum overload in the prenatal and perinatal periods," *World Journal of Pediatrics* 10 (2014): 101–107, https://link.springer.com/article/10.1007%2Fs12519-014-0477-x.

of this aluminum will enter and be stored in brain tissue. This aluminum may eventually be recruited to participate in toxicity in the body when the infant is an adolescent or a young adult or eventually at an indeterminate age to contribute toward neurological disease such as multiple sclerosis or Alzheimer's disease. Infant formulas are a surefire way to kick-start an individual's body burden of aluminum.

While I write these words about infant exposure to aluminum in the diet, I can almost feel the pressure from many readers asking, "But what about aluminum in vaccines?" Is there a more contentious subject in human health today than the safety of vaccines? Is there a subject laced with more vitriol? In the United Kingdom, the admission that you are researching vaccine safety is something akin to science heresy. If so, then I am proud to stand on the shoulders of past heretics like Galileo in my questioning the safety of the vaccines we administer to our children. I will not be bullied from doing so. Well, getting off my soapbox for a moment, I have written specifically about aluminum and vaccines elsewhere in this book, and I will simply emphasize here that which is important and specific to infants. Actually, as has already been implied, the unique vulnerability of infants to aluminum magnifies their predisposition to aluminum administered as an adjuvant in vaccines. The aluminum content of pediatric vaccines is absurdly high and a significant cause for concern.[11] Recall that vaccines requiring an aluminum adjuvant do not work in the absence of the adjuvant. The antigen is not by itself sufficiently antigenic to initiate any form of effective immune response. With this in mind, imagine the scene in the vaccine manufacturers' research laboratory at the time when they are testing the efficacy of a vaccine and, borrowing a term from the vaccine charlatan Andrew Pollard, its truly "minuscule" content (unlike the aluminum adjuvant) of antigen, to elicit the required antibody response. Every negative response is met with a war cry to increase the amount of aluminum adjuvant added to the vaccine until eventually an effective antibody titer is achieved. At no point does anyone in the research team question the significance of the amount of aluminum required to achieve the desired effect. There is no requirement to ask such a question. In spite of the obvious, that it is the aluminum adjuvant and not the vaccine per se that is immunoreactive, the adjuvant is considered as being benign in the process of development of the

11 Christopher Exley, "An aluminium adjuvant in a vaccine is an acute exposure to aluminium," *Journal of Trace Elements in Medicine and Biology* 57 (January 2020): 579–59, https://www.sciencedirect.com/science/article/pii/S0946672X19304201?via%3Dihub.

vaccine. There is no requirement in law to test the safety of the aluminum adjuvant alone,[12] and the safety of the whole vaccine is tested, nominally at least, against either the aluminum adjuvant or another vaccine that includes an aluminum adjuvant. Surely, *this* is "the dirty little secret" of vaccinology. When is a vaccine not a vaccine? When it doesn't contain an immunoreactive amount of aluminum adjuvant!

Manufacturers are at complete liberty to use as much aluminum adjuvant in a vaccine as befits their needs, in full knowledge that its toxicity will not be taken into account at any stage when the vaccine is tested for safety (cursory) and efficacy. This modern-day alchemy is behind the situation we have today where infants' major exposure to aluminum is from multiple vaccinations received during the first months, sometimes days, of their lives. That which I previously described herein as the intolerable scandal of aluminum exposure through infant formulas is surpassed by exposure through vaccination. Of course, most infants are receiving both, that is, daily chronic exposure through formula feeding and regular acute exposures through vaccinations. When aluminum is injected as an adjuvant in a vaccine, it is immediately inside the body. Thereafter it can only remain within the body or it can be excreted from the body, primarily in urine and sweat. The translocation of aluminum from the vaccine injection site involves a number of processes including its transport as complexes in blood and lymph and its transport within housekeeping, immunoreactive cells such as macrophages and lymphocytes (white blood cells).

Unlike the majority of aluminum that enters the bloodstream via the gut, aluminum from a vaccine will not pass through the liver, our major organ of detoxification, before having access to other major organs such as the heart and brain. Once again, returning to the thesis that the infant is an ideal laboratory model for aluminum intoxication, vaccination is the optimal route of exposure in such an ideal model. The infant is actually undergoing chronic, that is, day-to-day, intoxication by aluminum through diet, for example infant formula, and acute exposure to aluminum through vaccination. Human beings are robust, and infants are clearly no exception to this general rule. Wearing my toxicology hat, and remembering how aluminum killed fish, it is a wonder to me that more infants are not overtly

12 Emma Shardlow, Matthew Mold, and Christopher Exley, "Unraveling the enigma: elucidating the relationship between the physicochemical properties of aluminium-based adjuvants and their immunological mechanisms of action," *Allergy, Asthma & Clinical Immunology* 14 (November 7, 2018) https://aacijournal.biomedcentral.com/articles/10.1186/s13223-018-0305-2.

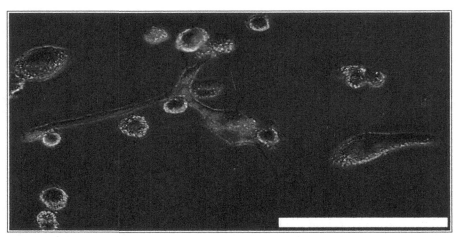

Figure 8. Aluminum-selective fluorescence microscopy showing aluminum adjuvant (orange fluorescence) inside a macrophage. Scale bar is 100μm. Please see the full paper for further information.** (See color version in insert.)

damaged by aluminum in their first few years of life. I emphasize, overtly, the covert damage suffered by infants from exposure to aluminum is only likely to manifest as chronic disease in adolescence and adulthood.

Of course, diet and vaccination are not the only ways in which infants are exposed to aluminum. Both over-the-counter and prescription medications including drugs such as antacids and painkillers are either aluminum-based or include aluminum salts as active ingredients. We used the General Practitioners Research Database (GPRD) in the United Kingdom to establish for any child up to the age of six if there was a link between prescription of an antacid and diagnosis of allergy. I was following a hunch that burgeoning childhood allergy was linked to increasing everyday exposure to aluminum. The result was unequivocal: any child prescribed an antacid was 69 percent more likely to be diagnosed with an allergy. This was only a look-and-see exercise and the results remain unpublished up until now, but it is an example of what we might expect for the health of children living in the Aluminum Age. Recently it was brought to my attention that aluminum salts are added to talc to help to produce the free-flowing friable

---

** Emma Shardlow, Matthew Mold, and Christopher Exley, "The interaction of aluminium-based adjuvants with THP-1 macrophages in vitro: Implications for cellular survival and systemic translocation," *Journal of Inorganic Biochemistry* 203 (February 2020) https://www .sciencedirect.com/science/article/pii/S0162013419305719?via%3Dihub.

product that is applied liberally to babies and self.[13] The question remains to be answered as to how this is adding to the body burden of aluminum in infants.

It is probably true that infants' relative exposure to aluminum in their everyday lives diminishes as they grow into older children and adolescents. However, processed foods that replace milk products as primary sources of infant nutrition are also contaminated with aluminum. Children's snacks and sweets are contaminated with aluminum. The use of aluminum lakes as colorings is rife in the food industry, and certain colored sweets, especially the blue and purple ones, are replete with aluminum. Every so often, a new piece of research relates children's sweets, usually interpreted as sugar uptake, to abnormal behavior such as Attention Deficit Hyperactivity Disorder (ADHD). The role that aluminum may play in this and other neurodevelopmental disorders of childhood remains to be determined through scientific study. Are conditions such as ADHD simply "mild" forms of more serious neurodevelopmental disorders such as autism?

The one certainty we have is that from before a child is born it is exposed to aluminum in myriad different ways, and that exposure continues from childhood into adolescence and onto adulthood. It is logical to my way of thinking that the earlier that this exposure begins and continues, the greater the likelihood of aluminum-related disease both immediately and later in life.

---

13 Cancer Corner USA home page, accessed September 30, 2020, http://cancercornerusa.com/.

CHAPTER 11

Tell Me Again Why There Is Aluminum in Vaccines

A life absorbed by the natural history of aluminum brought me only relatively recently into the field of vaccines. I had been aware for some time
of the seminal work of my great friend Romain Gherardi in Paris, the first
to show that an aluminum adjuvant in a vaccine was the cause of a specific disease. Macrophagic myofasciitis (MMF) was identified late in the
twentieth century by Gherardi as a condition relating to the persistence
of aluminum adjuvant at a vaccine injection site.[1] The etiology of MMF
is now known to be much more complex and manifests not only physi-
cally but mentally too, with significant neurological impairment. However,
at the time of Gherardi's seminal paper, the specific role of aluminum in
this disease did not register with me until several years later in 2008, when
I received a further prompt from an individual who had become severely
disabled immediately following injection of a suite of vaccines, each of
which included an aluminum adjuvant.[2] The individual had been obliged

1 R. K. Gherardi, M. Coquet, P. Cherin, L. Belec, P. Moretto, P. A. Dreyfus, J.-F. Pellissier, P.
   Chariot, and F.-J. Authier, "Macrophagic myofasciitis lesions assess long-term persistence of
   vaccine-derived aluminium hydroxide in muscle," *Brain* 124, no. 9 (September 2001): 1821–
   1831, https://academic.oup.com/brain/article/124/9/1821/303280.
2 Christopher Exley, Louise Swarbrick, Rhomain K. Gherardi, and Francois-Jérôme Authier,
   "A role for the body burden of aluminium in vaccine-associated macrophagic myofasciitis and
   chronic fatigue syndrome," *Medical Hypotheses* 72, no. 2 (February 2009): 135–139, https://
   www.sciencedirect.com/science/article/abs/pii/S0306987708004933?via%3Dihub.

to receive the vaccinations to enable him to take up a post supported by the Ministry of Defense in the United Kingdom. I put him in touch with Gherardi and Jerome Authier in Paris, where he was diagnosed as suffering from MMF. At Keele, we established by urinary aluminum excretion that he had a high body burden of aluminum. The previously fit individual who had been successfully employed as a photographer was forty-three years old at the time. Since receiving the vaccinations, he has not been able to work and has been forced to claim disability benefits, including from the Vaccine Damage Payments Unit run by the UK government.[3]

This seemingly extraordinary case prompted me to find an explanation for his terrible debilitating illness, and I raised a hypothesis to support a mechanism of immunological disease caused by aluminum adjuvants in vaccines. The hypothesis was built upon two important immunoreactive properties of aluminum; it was capable of acting as both adjuvant and antigen. The latter was perhaps considered the more novel of the two, though burgeoning research was already demonstrating that many different types of biologically reactive molecules, not just proteins, could act as antigens, aluminum included. Pioneers in demonstrating the antigenicity of aluminum is the group run by Beka Solomon in Tel Aviv, Israel, world leaders in antibody research. The notion that aluminum is an antigen means that the body retains a memory of previous exposures to aluminum. This means that any de novo exposure to aluminum might result in antibodies being raised not only against the new insult, but also against existing stores of aluminum in the body.

In brief, I suggested that the injection of five vaccines, each including an aluminum adjuvant, over just four weeks resulted in a highly immunogenic response in this individual. Recall that the aluminum content of each of these vaccines is optimized in development against the highest titer of antigen (not aluminum) antibodies considered safe. These optimizations do not take account of the antigenicity of aluminum. Titers for antibodies against aluminum in the vaccine are not measured. When an individual receives five aluminum adjuvant vaccines within a relatively short period of time, there is the potential for significant amplification of the aluminum antibody titer. At some point, perhaps following the second, third, fourth, or fifth vaccine, this amplification was sufficient to set off a cascade of immune responses including, potentially, against all of the aluminum already present

---

3 "Vaccine Damage Payment," Gov.uk, accessed September 30, 2020, https://www.gov.uk/vaccine -damage-payment/how-to-claim.

in the individual's body. The body burden of aluminum, and not just aluminum in the vaccine, becomes a target for attack by the immune system. The resulting antibody cascade would be capable of producing immediate and, in some tissues such as the brain, irreparable tissue damage. Only a mechanism so profound could explain the wholesale damage and illness experienced by this affected individual. Of course, aluminum, perhaps unlike a virus, cannot be neutralized by an antibody, and therein lies some of the issue and the long-term toxicity suffered by this individual. Antibody binding of extracellular aluminum may both liberate and redistribute aluminum in the body, changing, and possibly exacerbating, its propensity to bring about toxicity. We simply do not know if this is the case. The research into this hypothesized phenomenon has yet to be carried out. The perfect storm of toxicity in this individual was brought about because prior to receiving the five aluminum adjuvant vaccines in just four weeks, he already was subject to a higher than normal body burden of aluminum. The aluminum he received in the vaccinations was not sufficient in itself to explain his high body burden as measured by us postvaccinations at Keele. How, why, and when this body burden was built up is impossible to ascertain, but these previous exposures were sufficient to leave behind memories, antibodies primed for any future significant exposure to antigenic aluminum.

I emphasize significant exposure to aluminum, as aluminum is unlikely to be a potent antigen and the form of aluminum that is antigenic is almost certainly $Al^{3+}_{(aq)}$, which is present in the body at very low concentrations. This means that in practice, in normal daily life, only acute exposures to aluminum, as might be represented by a vaccine and certainly by five vaccines in just four weeks, will activate "aluminum the antigen" to raise an antibody response to proceed to address stores of aluminum throughout the body. In addition, the antibody response to an aluminum challenge will also need to be high for the antibodies to "find and bind" nanomolar concentrations of $Al^{3+}_{(aq)}$ in extracellular body stores and compartments.

Finally, it is worth noting that exposure to aluminum as an adjuvant does represent a form of exposure where high concentrations of $Al^{3+}_{(aq)}$ are possible. We know this from our research showing that aluminum adjuvant enclosed within membrane vesicles in the cytoplasm of immunoreactive cells gives an intense fluorescence, indicating the binding of $Al^{3+}_{(aq)}$ by the fluor lumogallion. What this means in essence is that the immunogenic response to stores of aluminum throughout the body is most likely to be initiated by an acute response to aluminum adjuvants. This potency of aluminum adjuvants is unlikely to be equaled by any other everyday exposure to aluminum. This mechanism proposed and published in 2009 remains to be tested in an experimental model. It would not be too onerous to compare how the body burden of aluminum in animal treatment groups impacts their response to multiple injections of an aluminum adjuvant vaccine.

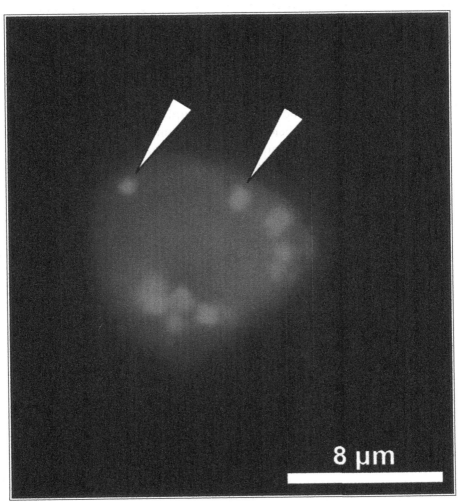

Figure 9. Aluminum-selective fluorescence microscopy showing aluminum adjuvant as orange fluorescence (white arrows) inside a T Helper 1 cell. Please see the full paper for further information.** (See color version in insert.)

** Matthew Mold, Håkan Eriksson, Peter Siesjö, Anna Darabi, Emma Shardlow, and Christopher Exley, "Unequivocal identification of intracellular aluminium adjuvant in a monocytic THP-1 cell line," *Scientific Reports* 4 (September 5, 2014) https://www.nature.com/articles/srep06287.

This unfortunate case, from the point of view of the affected individual, and the pioneering work of Romain Gherardi and his team in Paris opened my eyes and my mind to aluminum adjuvants as important pieces in the jigsaw puzzle that is human exposure to aluminum. A puzzle that is particularly pertinent today considering the burgeoning vaccine schedule with the majority of those vaccines including an aluminum adjuvant. We needed to know more, and it was clear from the published scientific literature that the great and the good of immunology did not understand why aluminum salts made such effective adjuvants. Paper after paper published in so-called high-esteem journals like *Nature* and *Science* showed a complete misunderstanding of the bioinorganic chemistry of aluminum. The majority of these papers reported research where the forms of aluminum salts used in experiments were not forms of aluminum used as clinical adjuvants in vaccines. They were making the scientifically naive assumption that all forms of aluminum salt were biologically equal. The authors of these flawed papers were not particularly open to my criticism of their methods. Fortunately, the editor of *Trends in Immunology* agreed with our reservations and published our opinion piece on how aluminum adjuvants "really" work.[4] While we did not know either at this time in 2010 how they "really" worked, writing the paper did give us the opportunity to delineate how one should go about investigating their actions in boosting the immune response. With this in mind, we began an active research program on aluminum adjuvants and succeeded in winning a research grant from the Medical Research Council (MRC) to investigate how aluminum adjuvants actually work. We surmised that by understanding their mode of action we would also get insight into why they were debilitating—toxic, in other words—in some individuals. We wanted to know why aluminum adjuvants were responsible for adverse events in some vaccinated individuals. Our research in this field over the past ten or so years has been extremely productive, and, in addition to providing full characterization of physical and chemical properties of aluminum adjuvants

4 Christopher Exley, Peter Siesjö, and Håkan Eriksson, "The immunobiology of aluminium adjuvants: how do they really work?" *Trends in Immunology* 31, no. 3 (March 1, 2010): 103–109, https://www.cell.com/trends/immunology/fulltext/S1471-4906(09)00248-8?_returnURL=https%3A%2F%2Flinkinghub.elsevier.com%2Fretrieve%2Fpii%2FS1471490609002488%3Fshowall%3Dtrue.

used in commercial vaccines,[5] it has also revealed critical information about their biology.[6]

It is of note that our successes in this field of vaccinology have been achieved in spite of an, at times, hostile and nonscientific backdrop of ill-found criticism. Rarely is this from fellow scientists; more often it is perpetrated by various press and social media outlets fueled by vaccine industry trolls. You can read more about this later in the book.

The biology of aluminum adjuvants and particularly at the vaccine injection site is dictated by their physical and chemical properties. Once these had been better understood, we were able to proceed to confirm unequivocally that particles of aluminum adjuvant are internalized by immunoreactive cells invading the vaccine injection site. This means that specific types of cells attracted to tissue damage occurring at the injection site literally eat aluminum adjuvant. However, they are fussy eaters; they seem to prefer to eat or bite off particles that are about one-thousandth of a millimeter in size. We know this because the "ingested" aluminum adjuvant is retained in the cytoplasm of invading cells within membrane-bound vesicles that are approximately one micron (1 μm) in diameter.[7] Here the aluminum adjuvant remains while the host cell is viable.[8] The fact that we can image the membrane-bound adjuvant with the fluor lumogallion tells us that the aluminum adjuvant salt is dissolving in the vesicle and releasing $Al^{3+}_{(aq)}$ to be bound by lumogallion. Membranous vesicles of this ilk are usually actively acidified by the cell as part of a mechanism of degradation—digestion—of their contents. The acidification begins to dissolve the particulate aluminum adjuvant. At some point, the concentration of $Al^{3+}_{(aq)}$ inside the structure will exceed a toxic threshold, and the endosome/lysosome/phagosome

5 Emma Shardlow, Matthew Mold, and Christopher Exley, "Unraveling the enigma: elucidating the relationship between the physicochemical properties of aluminium-based adjuvants and their immunological mechanisms of action," *Allergy, Asthma & Clinical Immunology* 14 (November 7, 2018) https://aacijournal.biomedcentral.com/articles/10.1186/s13223-018-0305-2.

6 Matthew Mold, Håkan Eriksson, Peter Siesjö, Anna Darabi, Emma Shardlow, and Christopher Exley, "Unequivocal identification of intracellular aluminium adjuvant in a monocytic THP-1 cell line," *Scientific Reports* 4 (September 5, 2014) https://www.nature.com/articles/srep06287.

7 Matthew Mold, Emma Shardlow, and Christopher Exley, "Insight into the cellular fate and toxicity of aluminium adjuvants used in clinically approved human vaccinations," *Scientific Reports* 6 (August 12, 2016) https://www.nature.com/articles/srep31578.

8 Emma Shardlow, Matthew Mold, and Christopher Exley, "The interaction of aluminium-based adjuvants with THP-1 macrophages in vitro: Implications for cellular survival and systemic translocation," *Journal of Inorganic Biochemistry* 203 (February 2020): 110915, https://www.sciencedirect.com/science/article/pii/S0162013419305719?via%3Dihub.

membrane surrounding the adjuvant will be compromised, releasing $Al^{3+}_{(aq)}$ into the parent cell cytosol. At this point, the cell may die either in a controlled manner called apoptosis or rapidly and violently through necrosis. Initially, cellular processes indicating the former may be instigated though the continued release of biologically reactive $Al^{3+}_{(aq)}$ will probably overwhelm many cells and necrotic death will ensue. Cell death via necrosis would allow cell contents, including any free or membrane-bound aluminum, to spill into the surrounding biological fluid, inducing, among a cascade of reactions, an inflammatory response. Necrotic cell death would also release sufficient quantities of $Al^{3+}_{(aq)}$ for it to act as an antigen in initiating an additional antibody response. We found clear evidence of necrotic cell death and concomitant inflammation in our seminal research on aluminum in brain tissue in autism.[9] What is concerning, therefore, and may be happening in serious adverse events brought about by vaccination is that cell death can occur anywhere in the body and not just at the vaccine injection site. We know this because cells loaded with membrane-bound aluminum adjuvant remain viable for days, at least, and in the case of macrophages, probably much longer; during this time they can translocate their cargos of aluminum to other tissues including the lymph[10] and brain tissue. Actually the stark realization that aluminum adjuvant might be transported from a vaccine injection site to the brain was brought to our attention in the aforementioned research on aluminum in human brain tissue in autism.

I am on record as saying that before the aforementioned research on autism I could not see an obvious link between human exposure to aluminum and autism.[11] In particular, it was difficult to reconcile the severely disabling form of autism in infants, often following vaccination, with aluminum toxicity. It was difficult because my understanding then on aluminum and the human brain was that before aluminum exerted toxicity it had to reach a toxic threshold in brain tissue, something I assumed would take years if not decades of continuous low-level exposure.[12] One early clue that aluminum

9 Matthew Mold, Dorcas Umar, Andrew King, and Christopher Exley, "Aluminium in brain tissue in autism," https://www.sciencedirect.com/science/article/pii/S0946672X17308763?via%3Dihub.

10 Javier Asín, Jéssica Molín, Marta Pérez, et al, "Granulomas Following Subcutaneous Injection With Aluminum Adjuvant-Containing Products in Sheep," *Veterinary Pathology* 56, no. 3 (May 1, 2019): 418–428, https://journals.sagepub.com/doi/10.1177/0300985818809142.

11 "Large doses of aluminum found in autistic brains," accessed October 1, 2020, https://www.youtube.com/watch?v=aS0cWQmQmLw.

12 Christopher Exley and Matthew J. Mold, "Aluminium in human brain tissue: how much

exposure through vaccination might be different came courtesy of a research collaboration with Romain Gherardi in Paris where it was shown in mice that intramuscular injection of aluminum and surrogate aluminum particles led to their subsequent presence in brain tissue.[13] While it was always assumed that the dissolution of aluminum adjuvant in the body would inevitably result in some aluminum entering brain tissue, this new research suggested that it could enter the brain as particulate aluminum. This highlighted a potentially faster way for larger amounts of aluminum to enter the brain. At about the same time as this new research was being published, I was asked by a vaccine court in Washington, DC, to elaborate upon the possibility that aluminum administered in a vaccine could be responsible for brain encephalopathy in an infant. Since aluminum-induced encephalopathy is widely known and accepted, for example in renal dialysis, the question critical to an infant became whether a high content of aluminum could be delivered into brain tissue within a relatively short time period. Our research, ongoing at the time, into the uptake of aluminum adjuvant by cells known to infiltrate vaccine injection sites suggested a mechanism. In the evidence I gave to the vaccine court, I described a scenario where an infant's brain signals a call for help, for example, due to a local inflammation. Housekeeping cells from the periphery, such as macrophages and lymphocytes, would answer the call by migrating into the brain across the blood-brain barrier and meninges. If these responding cells were loaded with aluminum, for example from a vaccine injection site, then this represented a mechanism whereby a high and toxic dose of aluminum might be delivered to a focal point in the brain. The inevitable subsequent death of these aluminum-loaded cells in brain tissue would release a highly toxic cargo of biologically reactive aluminum, producing further cell death of both neurones and nonneuronal cells. The resulting inflammation might then intensify the "help" signal to the body, bringing further potentially aluminum-loaded cells to the damaged tissue. These actions would result in an acute encephalopathy in the affected area of the brain. A feasible mechanism whereby vaccinations involving aluminum adjuvants might result in brain damage in an infant was, at that time, just that, a feasible mechanism.

---

is too much?" *Journal of Biological Inorganic Chemistry* 24 (August 29, 2019): 1279–1282, https://link.springer.com/article/10.1007%2Fs00775-019-01710-0.

13 Zakir Khan, Christophe Combadière, François-Jérôme Authier, Valérie Itier, François Lux, Christopher Exley, Meriem Mahrouf-Yorgov, Xavier Decrouy, Philippe Moretto, Olivier Tillement, Romain K. Gherardi, and Josette Cadusseau, "Slow CCL2-dependent translocation of biopersistent particles from muscle to brain," *BMC Medicine* 11 (April 4, 2013) https://bmcmedicine.biomedcentral.com/articles/10.1186/1741-7015-11-99.

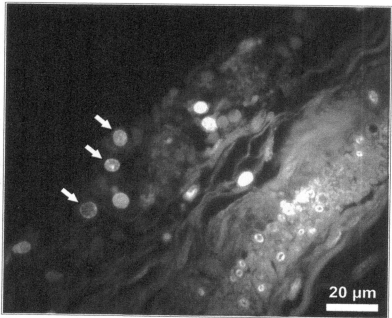

Figure 10. Aluminum-selective fluorescence microscopy showing lymphocytes loaded with aluminum (white arrows) crossing the meninges in brain tissue in autism. Please see the full paper for further information.** (See color version in insert.)

Our study on aluminum in brain tissue in autism provided the first direct evidence of such a mechanism.

The vaccine court case in Washington, DC, was one of a number of indirect prompts I received to investigate a role for aluminum in autism. Published science linked vaccines to autism, and several studies identified raised levels of aluminum in body fluids such as blood and urine in individuals with autism. We decided that if aluminum was involved, then we should expect to find it in brain tissue of people with autism. We contacted the Autism Brain Bank, part of the Oxford Brain Bank, and they had frozen tissue for five donors and fixed tissue for ten donors. Only deep-frozen tissue is suitable for quantitative determinations of aluminum. Fixed tissues, especially those preserved for some time, are prone to limited dissolution of aluminum from the tissue into the fixative.

There are certain moments as a scientist that always remain with you. One such moment happened a year before we did the autism measurements when

** Matthew Mold, Dorcas Umar, Andrew King, and Christopher Exley, "Aluminium in brain tissue in autism," *Journal of Trace Elements in Medicine and Biology* 46 (March 2018): 76–82, https://www.sciencedirect.com/science/article/pii/S0946672X17308763?via%3Dihub.

we got data on the extraordinarily high aluminum content in brain tissue in familial Alzheimer's disease.[14] We'll discuss this more later in the book. I was not expecting to be surprised again by the autism brain tissue, especially considering the young age of the donors. Yet the aluminum content of the brain tissue taken from donors who died with a diagnosis of autism was shockingly high. Shocking enough for me to pose the question in the published paper's abstract as to how a fifteen-year-old boy could have such a high amount of aluminum in his brain tissue.[15] However, while the quantity of aluminum was worryingly high, the location of aluminum in the tissues was revelatory. Actually, it was scary. In all ten cases we examined, the location of aluminum in the brain tissue was almost exclusively intracellular.

A predominance of intracellular aluminum was something we had not observed previously in, for example, Alzheimer's disease brain tissue. In addition, the types of cells where aluminum was predominantly found were nonneuronal cells, including microglia and cells resembling lymphocytes. Aluminum was largely identified in small punctate deposits in many of these cells, an observation that, you will recall, resembled closely how aluminum was found in immunoreactive cells known to populate vaccine injection sites. These small packets of intracellular aluminum were approximately 1 μm in diameter. Here in autism brain tissue was the first direct evidence to support the mechanism that had been proposed to the vaccine court. Was it possible that the very high content of aluminum in brain tissue in autism, where the majority of donors were adolescents and young adults, was the result of its translocation there by housekeeping cells, including lymphocytes and macrophages, from the peripheral circulation? Helper cells innocently carrying their cargoes of toxic aluminum into the brain both across the blood brain barrier and via the glymphatic system?

I presented this groundbreaking and thought-provoking research at a meeting in Paris in late November 2017.[16] I honestly expected to be spending the next days and weeks talking to the world's press about the research.

---

14 Ambreen Mirza, Andrew King, Claire Troakes, and Christopher Exley, "Aluminium in brain tissue in familial Alzheimer's disease," *Journal of Trace Elements in Medicine and Biology* 40 (March 2017): 30–36, https://www.sciencedirect.com/science/article/pii/S0946672X 16303777?via%3Dihub.

15 Mold, Umar, King, and Exley, "Aluminium in brain tissue in autism," *Journal of Trace Elements in Medicine and Biology*, https://www.sciencedirect.com/science/article/pii/S0946672 X17308763?via%3Dihub.

16 "Vaccinal aluminum could cause brain dysfunctions," accessed October 1, 2020, https:// www.youtube.com/watch?v=dLCFtqLBRQw&t=32s.

Autism donor			Total (T) number of intracellular (I) / extracellular (E) and gray matter (GM) brain regions			
			Frontal		Parietal	
Case	Age	Sex	WM	GM	WM	GM
A1	44	F	(I)1 (E)0 (T): 1	(I)0 (E)0 (T): 0	(I)0 (E)2 (T): 2	(I)0 (E)1 (T): 1
A6	29	F	N/A	N/A	(I)0 (E)0 (T): 0	(I)0 (E)0 (T): 0
A7	13	F	(I)0 (E)0 (T): 0	(I)0 (E)1 (T): 1	(I)1 (E)0 (T): 1	(I)0 (E)0 (T): 0
Female donor total			(I)1 (E)0 (T): 1	(I)0 (E)1 (T): 1	(I)1 (E)2 (T): 3	(I)0 (E)1 (T): 1
A2	50	M	(I)2 (E)0 (T): 2	(I)6 (E)0 (T): 6	(I)0 (E)2 (T): 2	(I)5 (E)5 (T): 10
A5	33	M	(I)0 (E)0 (T): 0	(I)0 (E)0 (T): 0	(I)0 (E)0 (T): 0	(I)0 (E)0 (T): 0
A8	29	M	(I)2 (E)1 (T): 3	(I)0 (E)0 (T): 0	(I)4 (E)0 (T): 4	(I)3 (E)1 (T): 4
A9	22	M	(I)0 (E)0 (T): 0	(I)1 (E)0 (T): 1	(I)0 (E)0 (T): 0	(I)2 (E)0 (T): 2
A3	22	M	(I)1 (E)2 (T): 3	(I)2 (E)0 (T): 2	(I)3 (E)2 (T): 5	(I)2 (E)1 (T): 3
A4	15	M	(I)1 (E)0 (T): 1	(I)2 (E)0 (T): 2	(I)1 (E)2 (T): 3	(I)2 (E)0 (T): 2
A10	14	M	(I)0 (E)0 (T): 0	(I)0 (E)0 (T): 0	(I)0 (E)0 (T): 0	(I)1 (E)0 (T): 1
Male donor total			(I)6 (E)3 (T): 9	(I)11 (E)0 (T): 11	(I)8 (E)6 (T): 14	(I)15 (E)7 (T): 22

Figure 11. Table identifying the location of aluminum deposits in brain tissue in autism. Please see the supplementary information in the full paper for further information.[**]

** Mold, Umar, King, and Exley, "Aluminium in brain tissue in autism," *Journal of Trace Elements in Medicine and Biology*, https://www.sciencedirect.com/science/article/pii/S0946672 X17308763?via%3Dihub.

Lumogallion-reactive aluminium deposits observed in white matter (WM) in male (M) and female (F) donors

Occipital		Temporal		Hippocampus	
WM	GM	WM	GM	WM	GM
(I)0 (E)3 (T): 3	(I)1 (E)2 (T): 3	(I)1 (E)0 (T): 1	(I)0 (E)3 (T): 3	(I)0 (E)0 (T): 0	(I)0 (E)0 (T): 0
N/A	N/A	N/A	N/A	(I)0 (E)0 (T): 0	(I)0 (E)1 (T): 1
(I)1 (E)3 (T): 4	(I)0 (E)0 (T): 0	N/A	N/A	(I)0 (E)0 (T): 0	(I)0 (E)0 (T): 0
(I)1 (E)6 (T): 7	(I)1 (E)2 (T): 3	(I)1 (E)0 (T): 1	(I)0 (E)3 (T): 3	(I)0 (E)0 (T): 0	(I)0 (E)1 (T): 1
(I)1 (E)0 (T): 1	(I)0 (E)4 (T): 4	(I)0 (E)0 (T): 0	(I)0 (E)3 (T): 3	(I)7 (E)0 (T): 7	(I)1 (E)2 (T): 3
(I)0 (E)0 (T): 0	(I)0 (E)0 (T): 0	(I)0 (E)0 (T): 0	(I)0 (E)0 (T): 0	(I)0 (E)0 (T): 0	(I)0 (E)0 (T): 0
(I)1 (E)0 (T): 1	(I)2 (E)0 (T): 2	N/A	N/A	(I)1 (E)0 (T): 1	(I)0 (E)0 (T): 0
(I)0 (E)1 (T): 1	(I)0 (E)0 (T): 0	(I)0 (E)0 (T): 0	(I)0 (E)0 (T): 0	(I)1 (E)0 (T): 1	(I)1 (E)0 (T): 1
(I)1 (E)1 (T): 2	(I)1 (E)0 (T): 1	(I)0 (E)1 (T): 1	(I)0 (E)1 (T): 1	(I)2 (E)3 (T): 5	(I)3 (E)1 (T): 4
(I)0 (E)1 (T): 1	(I)3 (E)0 (T): 3	(I)0 (E)0 (T): 0	(I)4 (E)0 (T): 4	(I)3 (E)0 (T): 3	(I)0 (E)0 (T): 0
(I)1 (E)0 (T): 1	(I)0 (E)1 (T): 1	(I)0 (E)2 (T): 2	(I)6 (E)1 (T): 7	(I)0 (E)0 (T): 0	(I)1 (E)1 (T): 2
(I)4 (E)3 (T): 7	(I)6 (E)5 (T): 11	(I)0 (E)3 (T): 3	(I)10 (E)5 (T): 15	(I)14 (E)3 (T): 17	(I)6 (E)4 (T): 10

Supplementary table 1. Summary table detailing the total number of lumogallion reactive deposits identified in human brain tissue, for 10 donors diagnosed with autism from the Oxford Brain Bank (OBB), UK. The total (T) number of intracellular (I) or extracellular (E) lumogallion-reactive aluminium deposits observed in white matter (WM) or gray matter (GM) brain regions in male (M) and female (F) donors are depicted.

Instead, I was hit by a wall of silence; the research was not covered by any form of mainstream media anywhere in the world. Media silence was quickly followed by a barrage of mindless and unscientific (nonsense and nonscience) criticism from Internet trolls and various media and industry stooges. In reality, not a single scientist of repute and knowledge has criticized the autism research either openly or directly to me. There have been no letters to the editor of the journal where the research was published pointing out flaws in methods or interpretation. The only scientists, though neither with any relevant expertise in the subject matter, criticizing the research in the media were two press stooges working for Buzzfeed, and neither of these had even read the paper.[17] Scientists in general can at least appreciate that, even if they do not accept their meaning, the data presented are irrefutable and robust and will remain so until challenged by equally reputable follow-up research. At the time of writing, they show that the aluminum content of brain tissue in autism is very high in every case of autism so far examined. The data, specifically the imaging, suggest that the origin of some of the aluminum is aluminum adjuvant from vaccination. A pressing question that remains is what is different about those infants that succumbed to disabling autism following vaccination? What is it about their physiology that predisposed them to accumulate high amounts of aluminum in their brain tissues at an early age? We asked a very similar question about aluminum and those who succumbed to familial Alzheimer's disease.

The use of aluminum salts as adjuvants in vaccines has a long history going back over one hundred years, and I have spoken about this history on numerous previous occasions.[18] I will not repeat this information herein. Instead, I will focus upon raising some further unknowns about aluminum adjuvants in vaccines. Of course, there is nothing inherently special about aluminum salts as adjuvants. There has been a process of natural selection ongoing through history resulting in aluminum salts being the adjuvant of choice. In comparison to other adjuvants, both historic and still in use today, aluminum salts are adjuvants of choice for a number of reasons.

1. They are sufficiently toxic, without being too toxic, at the vaccine injection site to be effective in boosting the immune response.

---

17 See Comment "Whither (Peer) Review of Science" at: https://www.hippocraticpost.com /infection-disease/aluminium-and-autism/, accessed October 1, 2020.

18 "Systemic Toxicity of Aluminium Adjuvants: Prof. Christopher Exley," accessed October 1, 2020, https://www.youtube.com/watch?v=GSgk5m3tds0&t=177s.

2. They are unregulated, which means that vaccine manufacturers can use as much aluminum in a vaccine as they require.
3. They are, as we say in England, "as cheap as chips," adding essentially no cost at all to that of a vaccine.
4. Above all, they appear to work, loosely defined, and almost no understanding of their modus operandi seems to be required by vaccine manufacturers or their regulators, our safety bodies, such as the FDA and the EMA. The old adage seems to apply: "if it ain't broke, don't fix it."

There is no requirement of vaccine manufacturers to demonstrate that aluminum adjuvants, the most critical component of this type of vaccine, are safe for use in humans. Consequently, there are no safety studies, and there are no aluminum adjuvants approved for use in human vaccines. Only whole vaccines including an aluminum adjuvant are tested to establish their efficacy and, often a secondary endpoint, safety for use in humans. However, the validity of safety tests, such as they are, for whole vaccines that include an aluminum adjuvant is brought into question when one considers that not a single aluminum adjuvant vaccine in use today has been tested against a true placebo or control.[19] Manufacturers have always chosen to test the efficacy (often couched as a safety trial) of a new aluminum adjuvant vaccine against either a previous vaccine that includes an aluminum adjuvant or, as is often the case, against the aluminum adjuvant alone. There is only one conceivable reason why they do this, and it is to cover up, or mask, the toxicity of aluminum adjuvants. They know that aluminum adjuvants are toxic both from their unpublished in-house work and from scarce published data. Regarding the latter, in the only example in the scientific literature of a whole aluminum adjuvant vaccine, Gardasil, being compared against a true placebo, saline, zero adverse events were recorded for the saline group, while both the whole vaccine and the adjuvant alone groups recorded identical incidences of adverse events of 2.4 percent. The stark reality of this vaccine is that for every one million recipients of a single injection of Gardasil, 24,000 are injured by the vaccine, and the majority of these injuries are almost certainly due to Merck's proprietary adjuvant, aluminum hydroxyphosphate sulphate. This adjuvant appears to be a sulphated version of the commercially available adjuvant

19 Christopher Exley, "Aluminium-based adjuvants should not be used as placebos in clinical trials," *Vaccine* 29, no. 50 (November 2011): 9289, https://www.sciencedirect.com/science/article/pii/S0264410X11013089?via%3Dihub.

aluminum hydroxyphosphate. However, Merck has repeatedly refused to make their adjuvant available for independent verification and testing.

Vaccine manufacturers do not deny that vaccines cause adverse (some very serious) events, since they list them on the vaccine patient information leaflet. They do so in full confidence that few (probably just a very small percentage) vaccine recipients or their representatives read this obligatory information. This situation is not improved by general practitioners and others administering vaccines failing to encourage recipients and caregivers to read the leaflet. While manufacturers may be abiding by national guidelines with respect to the safety of vaccines, they are wholly complacent by not attempting to improve the safety of their products. Indeed, why would they when governments consistently put out the "fake news" message that all vaccines are completely safe for everyone?[20] This wholly political message feeds the complacency of vaccine manufacturers and sustains a vicious and sometimes life-threatening circle of unnecessary toxicity for recipients. I am purposely saying "unnecessary" because only a lack of investment prevents vaccines from being much, much safer for all.

To borrow from Al Gore's "inconvenient truth," there is a convenient ignorance concerning the toxicity of aluminum that pervades the actions of immunologists, vaccinologists, and, most concerning of all, pediatricians administering vaccines. The use, perversely, of baby language to misinform individuals is rife and best exemplified by charlatans such as Andrew Pollard of the Oxford Vaccine Group informing the national press in the United Kingdom that "the amount of aluminum in a vaccine is minuscule." I have written extensively on the ridiculous stupidity of this comment, though it is unlikely to be a product of stupidity or even ignorance. It is the careful and directed use of a lie, information that quite rightly should be called "fake news."[21] As a scientist working on aluminum for almost four decades, I watched aluminum kill fish and witnessed its toxicity in trees and every example of animal model used in scientific research. I am relieved to say that I have not watched aluminum kill an infant, but I have no doubt that this is happening and that, in the majority of cases where this happens, the primary culprit is aluminum in vaccines. The late General Norman Schwarzkopf,

---

20 Professor Chris Exley, "Aluminium Adjuvants in Vaccines: Missing Information," *The Hippocratic Post*, December 2, 2019, https://www.hippocraticpost.com/pharmacy-drugs/aluminium-adjuvants-in-vaccines-missing-information/.

21 Christopher Exley, "An aluminium adjuvant in a vaccine is an acute exposure to aluminium," *Journal of Trace Elements in Medicine and Biology* 57 (January 2020): 57–59, https://www.sciencedirect.com/science/article/pii/S0946672X19304201?via%3Dihub.

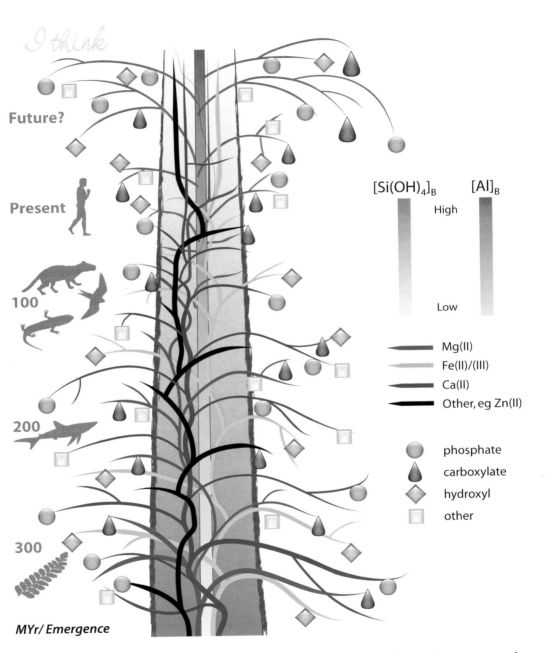

Here I have reimagined Charles Darwin's Tree of Life in order to demonstrate the emergence in evolutionary time of biologically reactive aluminum.

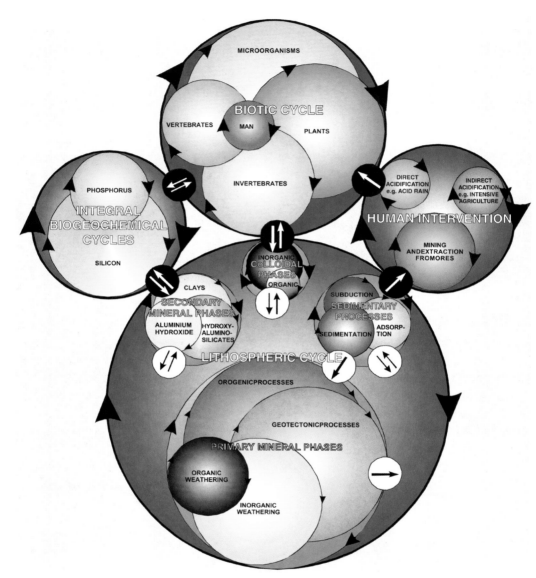

Aluminum's biogeochemical cycle ensured that almost no aluminum entered living things, the biotic cycle, until the advent of the Aluminum Age.

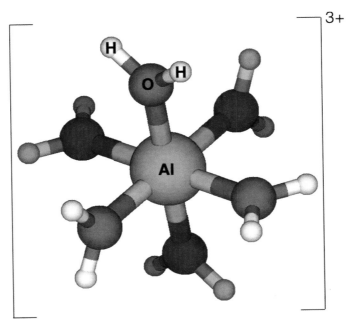

A model of biologically reactive aluminum. The aluminum atom is surrounded by six water molecules, giving an overall molecular charge of +3. *Courtesy of X. Lopez.*

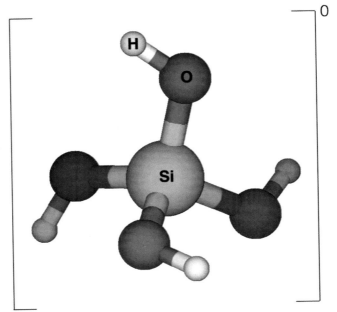

A model of silicic acid, the biologically available form of silicon. A central silicon atom is surrounded by four hydroxyl groups, giving an overall molecular charge of zero. *Courtesy of X. Lopez.*

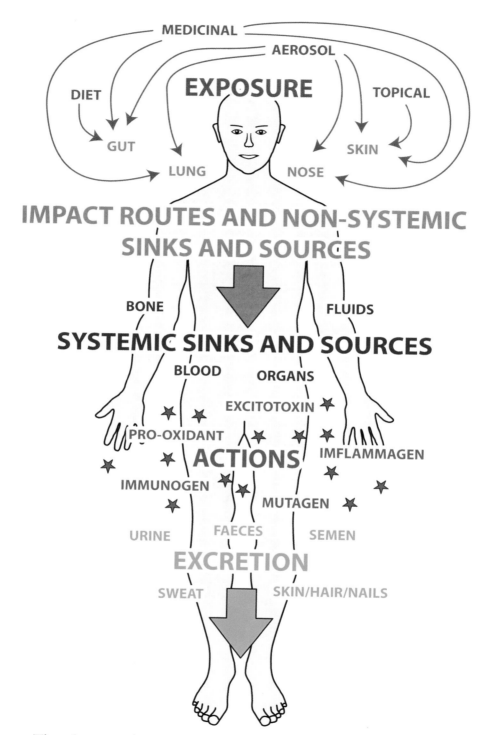

The schematic identifies the main factors, from uptake to excretion, involved with human exposure to aluminum.

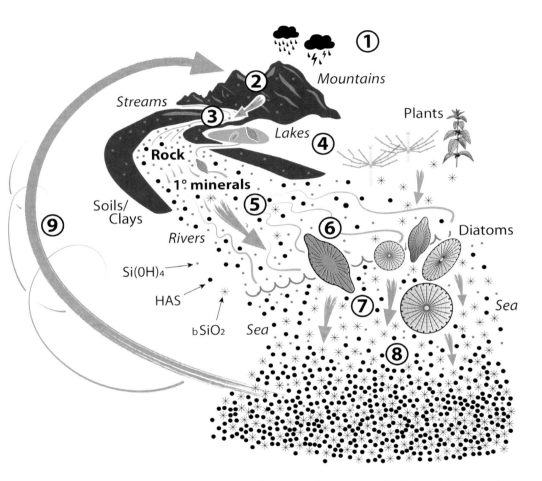

The schematic shows the silicic acid cycle from the formation of silicic acid through to its eventual deposition in sediments of rivers, lakes, and seas.

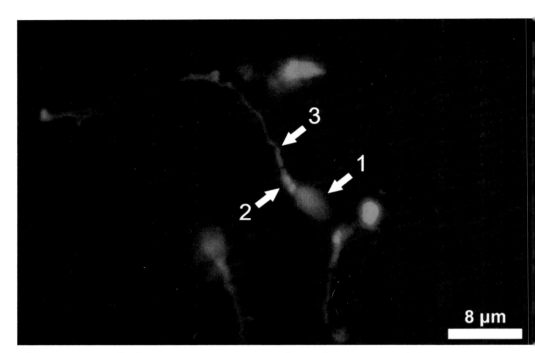

Aluminum-specific fluorescence microscopy shows the presence of aluminum as orange fluorescence in the head (1), midpiece (2), and tail of individual human sperm.

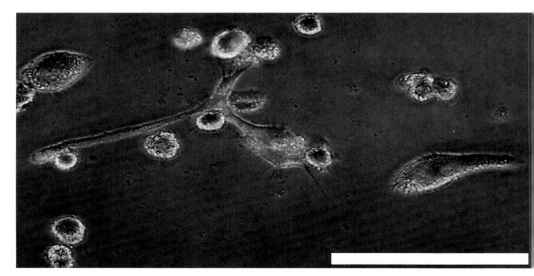

Aluminum-selective fluorescence microscopy showing aluminum adjuvant (orange fluorescence) inside a macrophage. Scale bar is 100μm.

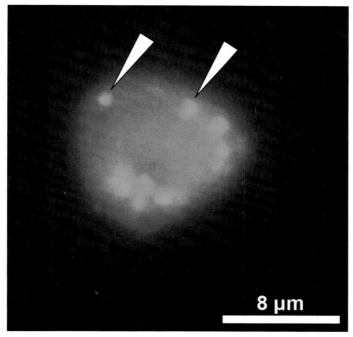

Aluminum-selective fluorescence microscopy showing aluminum adjuvant as orange fluorescence (white arrows) inside a T Helper 1 cell.

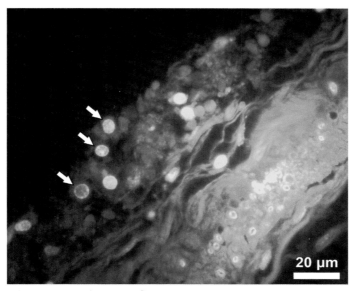

Aluminum-selective fluorescence microscopy showing lymphocytes loaded with aluminum (white arrows) crossing the meninges in brain tissue in autism.

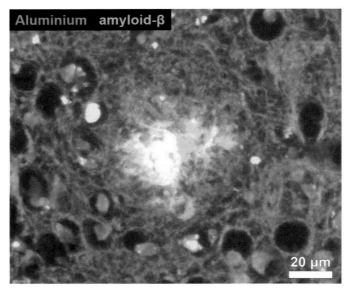

Fluorescence microscopy showing the colocation of aluminum (orange) and amyloid-β (green) in a senile plaque in brain tissue in Alzheimer's disease.

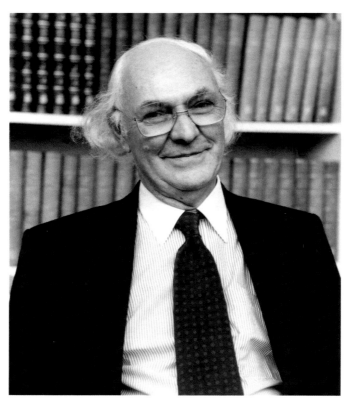

My "father-in-science," mentor, and great friend: the late JD Birchall OBE FRS.

better known as "Stormin' Norman," talked about collateral damage instead of referring directly to innocent people dying in the Gulf War. The collateral damage due to the use of aluminum adjuvants in infant vaccination is unnecessarily high, and until this is addressed, first by governments recognizing this and then by vaccine manufacturers, parents should think twice about vaccinating infants with any vaccine that includes an aluminum adjuvant. As a helpful rule, parents should ask themselves and their pediatrician a number of simple questions before submitting their child to a vaccine:

1. Is this a life-saving vaccine that has proven efficacy against a disease that my child is likely to encounter in everyday life?
2. Can vaccination be delayed, by months or even years, without putting my child in unnecessary harm?
3. Can the vaccination schedule be organized such that my child will not receive more than one aluminum adjuvant vaccine within a period of several months?

In addition, parents should ask to read the patient information leaflet in advance of a vaccination so that they can read about the vaccine and what it contains and understand about the known adverse events associated with it. The patient information leaflet includes information on the amount of aluminum in the vaccine. Different brands of vaccine use different amounts of aluminum adjuvant. Parents should choose the brand with the lowest stated aluminum content. At least until further research tells us otherwise. For example, future research may indicate that one form of aluminum adjuvant is less problematic than another and is therefore a possible lesser evil.

A combination of research and observational experience informs us that some individuals are more likely to suffer an adverse event following vaccination. Understanding of what it is that predisposes these individuals remains equivocal at time of writing, and the best advice is to avoid vaccination with an aluminum adjuvant if there is any history of autoimmune disease within the family. Include in this definition conditions such as allergy, eczema, and asthma. Another entirely unpredictable factor is our recent observation that the aluminum content of a vaccine given by the manufacturer on the patient information leaflet is typically incorrect. We have measured the aluminum content across several batches of many of the most common commercial vaccines and found that they vary significantly, even within the same batch. For example, within a pack of five ready-to-use vaccines, the aluminum content can vary by 50 percent or more. In many instances, the aluminum content is much higher than the amount stated in the patient information leaflet. This research will be published soon. This raises the possibility that adverse events might be more likely in those vaccinated with vaccines containing levels of aluminum exceeding the stated amount. However, to understand if this is possible, data relating to the safe level of aluminum adjuvant for a specific vaccine are required. How do manufacturers determine the aluminum content required for a vaccine? Upon which criteria are they basing the amount of aluminum stated on the patient information leaflet? There is little if any transparency in this area of vaccinology. We have visited this scenario previously in this book. However, a best guess is that manufacturers include an aluminum content that results in an optimal immune response, one that is deemed by their own standards to be both effective and safe. The safety of the vaccine presumably relates to the level of antigen antibodies produced as opposed to the direct toxicity of aluminum. Individual vaccines in which the aluminum content is above this optimal amount may instigate adverse events that relate to both the acuity of the immune response, a higher than optimal antibody titer, and additionally the direct toxicity of aluminum. It is, of course, impossible to know if this is the case, because either the requisite safety studies have not been carried out or the data from such studies are not in the public domain. We have asked the questions: Which concentration of aluminum adjuvant would produce a hyperactive immune response with concomitant adverse events? How often does this concentration of aluminum appear in a batch of vaccines?

We are beginning to understand the fundamental part played by aluminum adjuvants in vaccines, and, in doing so, we are also throwing light upon their safety and their role in vaccination-related adverse events. It is my opinion that prognoses for the future use of aluminum adjuvants in vaccines are decidedly gloomy. It is time to look elsewhere for effective and safe vaccines. There are, after all, alternatives to aluminum adjuvants already available[22] that are being routinely used in subcutaneous immunotherapy.[23]

---

22 Emma Shardlow and Christopher Exley, "The size of micro-crystalline tyrosine (MCT®) influences its recognition and uptake by THP-1 macrophages in vitro," *RSC Advances* 42 (2019): 24505-24518, https://pubs.rsc.org/en/content/articlelanding/2019/RA/C9RA03831K#!divAbstract.

23 Christopher Exley, "Aluminium adjuvants and adverse events in sub-cutaneous allergy immunotherapy," *Allergy, Asthma & Clinical Immunology* 10 (January 20, 2014) https://aacijournal.biomedcentral.com/articles/10.1186/1710-1492-10-4.

CHAPTER 12

Aluminum Is a Cause of and Contributor to Human Disease

So you think you are suffering from an aluminum-related disease. I have lost count of the number of times that someone has contacted me worried that they are suffering from some form of aluminum intoxication. With this in mind, my experience and understanding of living in the Aluminum Age tells me that the chances of being overloaded with aluminum are actually quite high. However, they also inform me that the likelihood of your being diagnosed as such, never mind being offered a treatment, is very poor.[1] "But, Dr. Exley, Professor, Chris, whatever," I hear you cry, "aluminum cannot be implicated in all human disease!"

Of course not, I tentatively reply, not ALL human disease. Over ten years ago, I attempted to square this circle in a book chapter I wrote called "Aluminum and Medicine"[2] by using the published scientific literature to produce a table of aluminum's likely role in human disease. I was looking into the future, and I hoped at the time that new research would subsequently confirm or refute my attempt at crystal ball gazing. In truth, new quality research directly relevant to aluminum and human health is still significantly lacking. However, I have now updated the table, and this has

---

1 C. Exley, "The toxicity of aluminium in humans/La toxicité de l'aluminium chez l'homme," *Morphologie* 100, no. 329 (June 2016): 51–55, https://www.sciencedirect.com/science/article/abs/pii/S1286011516000023.

2 Email me for a copy of the chapter.

DISEASE	RANKING 1 (low) – 10 (high)
Alzheimer's Disease	10
Parkinson's Disease	7-9
Motor Neurone Disease (MND/ALS)	4-6
Dialysis Encephalopathy	10
Multiple Sclerosis	8-10
Epilepsy	8-9
Osteomalacia	10
Osteoporosis	4-6
Arthritis	6-8
Anaemia	10
Calciphylaxis	2-4
Asthma	7-9
Chronic Obstructive Pulmonary Disease	6-8
Vaccine-related Macrophagic Myofasciitis	10
Vaccine-related Cutaneous Lymphoid Hyperplasia	8-10
Vaccine-related Hypersensitivity to Aluminium	8-10
Adverse Events following Vaccination	8-10
Immunotherapy-related Hypersensitivity to Aluminium	8-10
Adverse Events following Immunotherapy (SCIT)	8-10
Cancer	6-8
Diabetes	6-8
Sarcoidosis	7-9
Down's Syndrome	5-7
Muscular Dystrophy	4-6
Cholestasis	6-8
Obesity	5-7
Hyperactivity	5-7
Autism	7-9
Chronic Fatigue Syndrome	7-9
Gulf War Illness	6-7
Aluminosis	10
Crohn's Disease/IBD/UC	7-9
Vascular Disease / Stroke	6-8
Fertility/Reproduction	7-9
Breast Cancer	8-10
Autoimmune Conditions	7-9
Immunosuppression	7-10

Figure 12. Table depicting ranks for the involvement of aluminum in a number of human diseases.

not involved removing any disease conditions or downgrading any of their rankings.

If one aspect of such a table is abundantly clear, it is that aluminum writ large in the etiology of human disease is already a burgeoning pandemic. To employ the vernacular of the current day, self- or indeed forced isolation from this fact will not alone provide an inconvenient cure. To the contrary, it seems inevitable that more conditions will be added to the table and that the individual rankings of aluminum-related diseases will continue to rise. As I have written about elsewhere herein, the omnipresence of biologically reactive aluminum in the human body does implicate it in myriad human diseases. The human body continually reacts to its body burden of aluminum. If nothing else, this presents an energy deficit: the body uses energy that would otherwise be available for other roles. If I could remove all aluminum from my body, I would expect an overall increase in vitality. I would have more energy for other bodily functions and including those that protect me from disease. Therefore, the body burden of aluminum automatically increases your susceptibility to disease indirectly through affecting your energy currency and directly, for example, by suppressing your immune system. I trust the irony of the latter is not lost in considering the use of aluminum adjuvants in vaccines to boost the immune response.

I am often asked about synergistic reactions involving aluminum and other putative stressors including, for example, heavy metals like mercury. In biology and medicine, the term synergistic implies an overall effect that is greater than the sum of the individual parts. This would be the case where the nonredox metal aluminum acts as a prooxidant catalyzing oxidative damage initiated by, for example, redox active iron.[3] However, it would not be so where both aluminum and mercury bring about toxicity in a cell through completely independent mechanisms, the latter reflecting the "chalk-and-cheese" differences in these two metals' bioinorganic chemistries. Yes, aluminum is a stressor, and we know from the seminal work of Hans Selye that stress effects are cumulative but not necessarily synergistic.[4] There are myriad stressors acting upon our bodies all of the time, and when the outcome

3 J. I. Mujika, F. Ruipérez, I. Infante, J. M. Ugalde, C. Exley, and X. Lopez, "Pro-oxidant Activity of Aluminum: Stabilization of the Aluminum Superoxide Radical Ion," *Journal of Physical Chemistry A* 115, no. 24 (May 23, 2011): 6717–6723, https://pubs.acs.org /doi/10.1021/jp203290b.

4 Siang Yong Tan, MD, and A Yip, MS, "Hans Selye (1907–1982): Founder of the stress theory," *Singapore Medical Journal* 59, no. 4 (April 2018): 170–171, https://www.ncbi.nlm.nih .gov/pmc/articles/PMC5915631/.

is our overall health, these agents rarely act either truly independently or, importantly, synergistically. The fact that aluminum is a metallic element is often confusing for many. In the main, there is no metallic aluminum in your body. The exceptions are its rare use in various implants. So, when thinking about the toxicity of aluminum and perhaps any interactions or synergisms with other agents, for example, electromagnetic radiation, you do not need to consider metallurgy. As I have said earlier in the book, the toxic form of aluminum in the body is its free metal cation, $Al^{3+}_{(aq)}$.

The purpose of publishing herein an upgrade of aluminum's league table of disease is not to examine the minutiae of aluminum's putative role in each of the mentioned conditions. This would represent a Herculean task and I am not convinced that any of us would be any the wiser for my attempting such a task. However, a number of specific diseases and conditions, for which new data are currently burgeoning, will be covered in detail in following chapters. My intention is that the table act as a historical record and a signpost of a possible future. I have written on more than one occasion about the difficulty of obtaining a diagnosis by a physician of aluminum intoxication.[5] Your general practitioner or consultant is not well placed to make such a diagnosis. However, they may independently diagnose you with one of the conditions listed in the table, and you might then, reflecting upon your own personal environment, consider if aluminum could be playing a role. You can make an informed opinion and suggest to your medical practitioner that your exposure to aluminum might be involved and that measurement of your body burden of aluminum should be a next step. The table is science-based, and it can empower you to implicate aluminum where such a diagnosis would not be made by the regular medical establishment. There is a burgeoning number of common medical conditions that even your run-of-the-mill general practitioner should now be linking to your exposure to aluminum. Let us now have a more detailed look at some of them.

---

5 Christopher Exley, "The toxicity of aluminium in humans/La toxicité de l'aluminium chez l'homme," *Morphologie*, https://www.sciencedirect.com/science/article/abs/pii/S1286011516000023.

CHAPTER 13

What We Need to Know about Aluminum in Human Brain Tissue

We have measured the concentration of aluminum in over two hundred human brains.[1] This equates to several thousand individual tissue samples. We have applied the same method involving the same quality assurance criteria to measure each sample of tissue.[2] This extraordinary attention to detail has allowed us to make genuine and robust comparisons between data from tissues originating from donors who died with diagnoses of Alzheimer's disease, Parkinson's disease,[3] multiple sclerosis, autism, epilepsy, cancer, and representative control groups. The latter includes an age- and gender-matched control group for multiple sclerosis[4] and a large control group chosen specifically by the London Brain Bank to include only

1 Professor Christopher Exley, "Aluminium in human brain tissue," *The Hippocractic Post*, May 8, 2020, https://www.hippocraticpost.com/pharmacy-drugs/aluminium-in-human-brain-tissue/.

2 Emily House, Margaret Esiri, Gill Forster, Paul G Ince, and Christopher Exley, "Aluminium, iron and copper in human brain tissues donated to the medical research council's cognitive function and ageing study," *Metallomics* 1 (2012) https://pubs.rsc.org/en/content/articlelanding/2012/MT/C1MT00139F#!divAbstract.

3 Research in progress.

4 C. Linhart, D. Davidson, S. Pathmanathan, T. Kamaladas, and C. Exley, "Aluminium in Brain Tissue in Non-neurodegenerative/Non-neurodevelopmental Disease: A Comparison with Multiple Sclerosis," *Exposure and Health* (February 25, 2020) https://link.springer.com/article/10.1007%2Fs12403-020-00346-9.

individuals who died showing neither signs of neurological impairment nor neurodegenerative disease.[5] It has often bemused and frustrated me in equal amounts that publication of our data on, for example, aluminum in brain tissue in Alzheimer's disease has been met with criticism, valid under "normal" experimental rules, that they are not compared with "control" brain tissue. I am bemused because such a suggestion implies that the presence of aluminum, a known neurotoxin, in brain tissue is normal. I am hoping that by reaching this part of the book, the reader can already agree with me that there is absolutely nothing normal about having aluminum in your brain. I have written quite extensively about what might constitute control brain tissue for comparison with aluminum-related diseases, and one can quickly come to a conclusion that these ideal brain donors are few and far between.[6] Critics—might I suggest the armchair version—of research on human brain tissue react in a manner befitting what one might expect for research involving animal models. They quickly forget or probably misunderstand the difficulties in obtaining such privileged tissues. You do not allow yourself to forget this when you have human brain tissue under your scalpel in the laboratory. Those individuals who donate their brains for medical research are very special, and we are all indebted to them. However, such voluntary acts of benevolence dictate the brain tissues available, and as scientists, we can only work with donated tissues. The control brain tissues that we have measured are telling us one thing consistently, and this is that individual donors with low amounts of aluminum in their brain tissue did not die with a diagnosis of Alzheimer's disease, Parkinson's disease, multiple sclerosis, or autism.

5 Christopher Exley and Elizabeth Clarkson, "Aluminium in human brain tissue from donors without neurodegenerative disease: A comparison with Alzheimer's disease, multiple sclerosis and autism," *Scientific Reports* 10 (May 8, 2020) https://www.nature.com/articles/s41598-020 -64734-6.

6 Christopher Exley and Matthew J. Mold, "Aluminium in human brain tissue: how much is too much?" *Journal of Biological Inorganic Chemistry* 24 (August 29, 2019): 1279–1282, https:// link.springer.com/article/10.1007%2Fs00775-019-01710-0.

CHAPTER 14

Alzheimer's Disease and the Aluminum Elephant in the Room

Not everyone is entirely sure why he or she threw away their pots and pans made out of aluminum, but at that time they probably thought that it had something to do with Alzheimer's disease. In a game of word association, aluminum will often elicit Alzheimer's disease as a reply, though the reverse—aluminum as a reply to Alzheimer's disease—is far less likely. Nevertheless, the connection runs deep and is significant enough for manufacturers of said pots and pans to have changed their composition (to an anodized, hardwearing form of aluminum) to reduce loss of aluminum to food during cooking. However, while these changes in everyday use of aluminum are evident on the high street, large retailers furnishing organizations such as schools and hospitals still sell "old-style" aluminum pots and pans. It would seem that our children and hospitalized populations still receive their daily doses of aluminum from cooking pots, pans, and utensils. Manufacturers and retailers responded to public concerns by making visible changes to products sold on the high street while continuing to supply cheap and harmful products under the cover of hidden kitchens in most public institutions. Something akin to out of sight, into the mind! The availability of aluminum pots and pans is an allegory of the aluminum industry's complacency toward human exposure to aluminum and, perhaps specifically, Alzheimer's disease. This decision by the aluminum industry to continue to expose the most vulnerable in society, children and the hospitalized, to aluminum is, at best, complacent, while, in another example, the inclusion of aluminum as a listed ingredient in the Alzheimer's disease drug, Reminyl, is simply criminal. Imagine the behind-the-scenes discussions at the drug's manufacturer, Janssen-Cilag, about using an aluminum dye to give their flagship Alzheimer's disease drug a yellow appearance. It is probably the "company joke." Their inclusion of aluminum in a drug, Reminyl, that has no proven benefit in Alzheimer's disease in full knowledge of (if nothing else) a link between aluminum and the disease is, as I have said, nothing short of a crime against humanity. One day, perhaps soon, when the lawyers get hold of this information, the joke will be on Janssen-Cilag.

There are good reasons why people threw away their aluminum pots and pans, and these are all very much science-based.[1] The recent history of a link between aluminum and Alzheimer's disease goes back at least fifty years, while the first suggestions that exposure to aluminum was "bad for the brain" were made a century ago, about twenty years into the Aluminum Age. At about the same time, Alois Alzheimer reported the first case of the disease.[2] We now know that this case, a fifty-six-year-old woman, had familial Alzheimer's disease, and, as we will learn more about later in this chapter, given the opportunity to look, we would expect her brain tissue to be replete with aluminum.

The first compelling evidence in humans of a role for aluminum in Alzheimer's disease showed specific associations between aluminum and the two preeminent neuropathologies of the disease, neurofibrillary tangles and senile plaques. Supporting research confirmed the neurotoxicity of aluminum in both cell culture and animal models. Any doubts remaining about the neurotoxicity of aluminum in humans were dispelled with the advent of dialysis encephalopathy. When individuals with compromised kidney function underwent dialysis using tap water containing high concentrations of aluminum, a brain disorder characterized by widespread encephalopathy rapidly developed and progressed. Many died following dialysis, and analyses of their brain tissues showed high levels of aluminum.[3] This iatrogenic condition was

1 Christopher Exley, "Why industry propaganda and political interference cannot disguise the inevitable role played by human exposure to aluminum in neurodegenerative diseases, including Alzheimer's disease," *Frontiers in Neurology* 27 (October 2014) https://www.frontiersin.org /articles/10.3389/fneur.2014.00212/abstract.

2 Ulrich Müller, Pia Winter, and Manuel B Graeber, "A presenilin 1 mutation in the first case of Alzheimer's disease," *The Lancet Neurology* 12, no. 2 (February 1, 2013): 129–130, https://www .thelancet.com/journals/laneur/article/PIIS1474-4422(12)70307-1/fulltext.

3 Christopher Exley, "What is the risk of aluminium as a neurotoxin?" *Expert Review of Neurotherapeutics* 14, no. 6 (April 30, 2014): 589–591, https://www.tandfonline.com/doi/full /10.1586/14737175.2014.915745.

only resolved when dialysis centers changed to using pure water in dialysis, and even then, the additional use of aluminum salts as phosphate binders in the gut prolonged the problems and, in less severe cases, heralded a number of novel aluminum-related conditions such as the bone disease osteomalacia and a non-iron-responsive form of anemia. The latter has a familiar ring about it in these current days of COVID-19 infections. The lessons from dialysis encephalopathy are clear in demonstrating the rapid movement of aluminum from blood to brain and the immediate neurotoxicity of aluminum entering the brain. Not everyone suffering encephalopathy died: some survived following treatment with desferrioxamine (DFO), a known chelator of aluminum and iron. Thus, the removal of aluminum from the body prevented further neurotoxicity, and, while not reversing the damage done, it confirmed aluminum as the toxin responsible for dialysis-related encephalopathy. While dialysis encephalopathy is now largely confined to history, it is all the affirmation needed of the neurotoxicity of aluminum in humans.

Why then is there so much heated opposition to a role for aluminum in Alzheimer's disease? The scientific evidence is overwhelming and the equal of any other single contributory factor in Alzheimer's disease etiology. I have argued previously that the reasons why aluminum is so easily discounted can only be political. The largest "noises" in this discussion come from disciples of the aluminum industry. I have called them the aluminum ambassadors, and they are invariably scientists with strong reputations working in the field of Alzheimer's disease who have accepted the forty pieces of silver that are always on offer.[4] They include such distinguished scientists as the late Henryk Wisniewski, a prominent Alzheimer's researcher in the United States, and, in the United Kingdom, James Edwardson and Carol Brayne both occupied the position of chief scientific advisor to the Alzheimer's Society. It is no wonder that this so-called charity has never funded any research on aluminum and Alzheimer's disease. This pharmaceutical industry-funded organization actually actively campaigns against a role for aluminum, calling it an urban myth on their website. I am sure that the many people who actively campaign on behalf of this Janus charity are completely unaware of its links to the aluminum industry. The majority of scientists working in Alzheimer's disease and related fields do not have an informed

---

4 Christopher Exley, "Why industry propaganda and political interference cannot disguise the inevitable role played by human exposure to aluminum in neurodegenerative diseases, including Alzheimer's disease," *Frontiers in Neurology*, https://www.frontiersin.org/articles/10.3389/fneur.2014.00212/full.

opinion on whether or not aluminum is involved in the disease. They are taking advice from the aluminum ambassadors, as do all grant-giving bodies and most high-profile journals, and they repeat dogma fed to them and to all who will listen. I have literally lost count of the number of times that a reviewer of a manuscript or grant application has written that a link between aluminum and Alzheimer's disease was disproven years ago.

There are many forces working to undermine anything and everything that purports to link human exposure to aluminum with Alzheimer's disease. They have been successful in suppressing research and preventing reporting of research in so-called high-esteem journals. They ensure that there is no discussion of aluminum and Alzheimer's in mainstream media. The propaganda machine of the aluminum industry is all-powerful and malevolent. It has recruited most major industries and governments around the world to its cause. However, it has not silenced "the people," and the potent combination of social media and philanthropy has ensured the continuation of seminally important research into aluminum and Alzheimer's disease. Fortunately, there also remain editors-in-chief of reputable journals who are not cowed into rejecting such research without peer review, and the science is now clear, if still ignored, that aluminum is a cause of Alzheimer's disease.[5]

Previously I have brought together the entirety of the evidence that now supports human exposure to aluminum as a cause of Alzheimer's disease,[6] and herein I will only discuss the latest research affirming this conclusion. Historically, the aluminum industry was in perpetual denial that aluminum is present in human brain tissue. They repeated the common and convenient delusion that aluminum identified by any means in brain tissue was due to issues of contamination. Aluminum as the universal contaminant was their rallying call. They even recruited the Wellcome Trust and some University of Oxford academics and colluded with the journal *Nature* to publish so-called research that appeared to confirm their view on contamination. One of those Oxford scientists, the late and great RJP Williams FRS, was not prepared to go along with what would now be called "fake news" and withdrew his name from the manuscript prior to its being submitted.

5 Matthew Mold, Caroline Linhart, Johana Gómez-Ramírez, Andrés Villegas-Lanau, and Christopher Exley, "Aluminum and Amyloid-β in Familial Alzheimer's Disease," *Journal of Alzheimer's Disease* 73, no. 4 (February 18, 2020): 1627–1635, https://content.iospress.com /articles/journal-of-alzheimers-disease/jad191140.

6 Christopher Exley, "Aluminum Should Now Be Considered a Primary Etiological Factor in Alzheimer's Disease," *Journal of Alzheimer's Disease Reports* 1, no. 1 (June 8, 2017): 23–25, https://content.iospress.com/articles/journal-of-alzheimers-disease-reports/adr170010.

He, like myself, had been present at the 1992 Ciba Foundation Symposium on Aluminum in Biology and Medicine, where the shortcomings of the method behind the soon thereafter to-be-published research were discussed in detail. Williams expressed his reservations to his Oxford colleagues, and despite his significant seniority, his views were ignored. Other forces above and beyond science were determined to see this research published in science's premier journal.[7] *Nature* allowed very little criticism of this paper in their correspondence section. The paper was extremely damaging and put paid-to research into aluminum and Alzheimer's disease. A situation that persists to this day.

We addressed the criticism of "universal contamination" in our seminal study, funded by Somerset County Council (see the upcoming chapter on Camelford) that looked at the aluminum content of sixty human brains.[8] In this study, all issues of potential contamination were addressed, from the moment of collection of tissues at the brain bank at the University of Sheffield to the measurement of their aluminum content at Keele University. In addition to all the usual quality assurance criteria associated with such procedures and measurements, we also prepared over one hundred method blanks to assess the possibility of adventitious contamination of samples. These method blanks gave us a quantitative expression of worst-case contamination, and this value was then subtracted from all tissue values measured thereafter. We also measured total iron and copper in these method blanks, and these data helped to dispel the aluminum industry myth that aluminum was the universal contaminant. Our data showed that contaminating levels of iron and copper were significantly higher than for aluminum. Perhaps needless to say, our research proved beyond all doubt that human brain tissue contained significant amounts of aluminum. The relationship between the amount of aluminum in brain tissue and disease was addressed through the development of an imaging technique for the unequivocal identification of aluminum in human brain tissue: a method to see aluminum in human brain tissue.[9] We used this armory of complemen-

---

7 J. P. Landsberg, B. McDonald, and F. Watt, "Absence of aluminium in neuritic plaque cores in Alzheimer's disease," *Nature* 360 (November 5, 1992): 65–68, https://www.nature.com/articles/360065a0.

8 House, Esiri, Forster, Ince, and Exley, "Aluminium, iron and copper in human brain tissues donated to the medical research council's cognitive function and ageing study," *Metallomics*, https://pubs.rsc.org/en/content/articlelanding/2012/MT/C1MT00139F#!divAbstract.

9 Ambreena Mirza, Andrew King, Claire Troakes, and Christopher Exley, "The Identification of Aluminum in Human Brain Tissue Using Lumogallion and Fluorescence Microscopy," *Journal of Alzheimer's Disease* 54, no. 4 (October 18, 2016): 1333–1338, https://content.iospress.com /articles/journal-of-alzheimers-disease/jad160648.

tary quantitative and qualitative methods to measure and locate aluminum in brain tissue in Alzheimer's disease, autism, multiple sclerosis, epilepsy, and, currently, once they let us back into the laboratory, Parkinson's disease.

However, despite our seminal study on sixty human brains, resistance to a role for aluminum in Alzheimer's disease has reached legendary proportions to the extent that, as previously stated, Alzheimer's disease charities now actively campaign against any such possibility. We looked to address this continued resistance by carrying out what should have been the definitive study. The majority of research and researchers in Alzheimer's disease postulate that something called the Amyloid Cascade Hypothesis underlies the disease. This hypothesis puts the deposition of a small peptide, amyloid-β, in brain tissue as the principal tenet underlying Alzheimer's disease. Strong support for this view is the occurrence of early onset Alzheimer's disease in individuals carrying genetic predispositions that increase the production of amyloid-β in brain tissue. Quite simply, these genetic traits bring about the onset of Alzheimer's disease at age forty or fifty as opposed to seventy or eighty in the normal, common form (often referred to as sporadic) of the disease.

We speculated that individuals who died with a diagnosis of familial Alzheimer's disease, possessing these genetic predispositions, would, similarly to sporadic Alzheimer's disease and in spite of their much younger age range, have a high content of brain aluminum. What we actually found was remarkable: not just a high content, but some of the highest concentrations of aluminum ever measured in human brain tissue.[10] At the time of publication of the study, late 2016, these surprising—even horrifying—data, combined with images of aluminum in brain tissue, elicited almost no interest in mainstream media. I recall that on the day that our research was published, there was a story on the late evening news about how far you lived from a main road might influence your chance of having Alzheimer's disease in later life. This, not our research, was the big health news story of the day. The propaganda machinery of the aluminum industry and their disciples such as the Alzheimer's Society were making sure that aluminum and Alzheimer's disease remained securely in the realm of myth. While such propaganda and wholesale blocking, perhaps blacklisting, of published

10 Ambreen Mirza, Andrew King, Claire Troakes, and Christopher Exley, "Aluminium in brain tissue in familial Alzheimer's disease," *Journal of Trace Elements in Medicine and Biology* 40 (March 2017): 30–36, https://www.sciencedirect.com/science/article/pii /S0946672X16303777?via%3Dihub.

research does not change the science, it can and does make future research on the subject more difficult.

However, undaunted, we looked to Colombia in South America, where a brain bank had tissues from a famous cohort of familial Alzheimer's disease. Surely, these brains would not be characterized by the very high levels of aluminum found in the London Brain Bank cohort, would they? Remarkably, they were just as high in aluminum, and, added to this, we made the equally profound observation that aluminum was invariably colocated with amyloid-β in these tissues.[11] There was an intimate relationship between aluminum and amyloid-β in all of the cases of Colombian familial Alzheimer's disease. It was surely not a coincidence that different cohorts of familial Alzheimer's disease thousands of miles, indeed oceans and cultures, apart had very high levels of aluminum in their brain tissues. Nor, it would seem, was it coincidental that aluminum was an integral part of the amyloid cascade hypothesis in these individuals.[12] As I mentioned earlier in this chapter, the first reported case of Alzheimer's disease was familial and occurred within two decades of the advent of the Aluminum Age. This is also an unlikely coincidence. In 1906, the nascent Aluminum Age was too young to be responsible for late onset, sporadic Alzheimer's disease. At the turn of the twentieth century, only individuals who were predisposed to the accumulation and retention of aluminum in brain tissue would be susceptible to Alzheimer's disease. Sporadic Alzheimer's disease, in the absence of such predispositions, would result following near-lifelong living in the Aluminum Age.

We published this follow-up groundbreaking research on familial Alzheimer's disease, described as a landmark study by journal Editor-in-Chief George Perry, in the *Journal of Alzheimer's Disease* in January 2020, and waited for the mountains of opposition to aluminum as an etiological factor in Alzheimer's disease to crumble. We are still waiting. Indeed, the media blackout that followed the first paper was even more complete for the new study, and we did not receive any interest from any mainstream media outlet. This is science that, thirty years ago, would have been featured on

11 Mold, Linhart, Gómez-Ramírez, Villegas-Lanau, and Exley, "Aluminum and Amyloid-β in Familial Alzheimer's Disease," *Journal of Alzheimer's Disease*, https://content.iospress.com /articles/journal-of-alzheimers-disease/jad191140.

12 Christopher Exley and Matthew J. Mold, "Imaging of aluminium and amyloid β in neurodegenerative disease," *Heliyon* 6, no. 4 (April 1, 2020): E03839, https://www.cell .com/heliyon/fulltext/S2405-8440(20)30684-8.

every news channel across the globe. The fact that it did not is testimony to the power of the aluminum industry.

I am convinced that aluminum is a cause of Alzheimer's disease and that if there were no aluminum in the brain, there would be no Alzheimer's disease within a human lifespan of at least one hundred years. While published research in this field over recent decades is scant—after all, where there is no funding there is concomitantly no research—the research that has been carried out supports my view. However, the definitive proof could come from an appropriate clinical trial involving several hundred participants. For example, we know that a significant proportion of individuals diagnosed with mild cognitive impairment (MCI) go on to develop full-blown Alzheimer's disease. If individuals, upon being diagnosed with MCI,

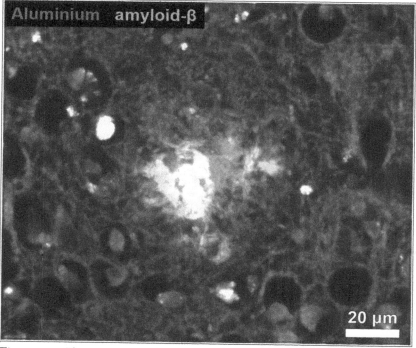

Figure 13. Fluorescence microscopy showing the colocation of aluminum (orange) and amyloid-β (green) in a senile plaque in brain tissue in Alzheimer's disease. Please see full paper for further information.** (See color version in insert.)

** Mold, Linhart, Gómez-Ramírez, Villegas-Lanau, and Exley, "Aluminum and Amyloid-β in Familial Alzheimer's Disease," *Journal of Alzheimer's Disease*, https://content.iospress.com/articles/journal-of-alzheimers-disease/jad191140.

were put onto a regimen that is known to limit their exposure to aluminum, then it could be determined if such a regimen delayed or prevented the onset of Alzheimer's disease. Living in the Aluminum Age does not make adopting such a regimen a trivial task. However, it is possible. If all recruited individuals are monitored over, for example, three to five years, it could be ascertained through regular urine sampling if their everyday exposure to aluminum was reduced and if this provided any benefit with respect to the development of Alzheimer's disease. I have written about the nature of a regimen in which a low exposure to aluminum could be achieved in Chapter 9. However, you will probably already have surmised that it includes regular drinking of silicon-rich mineral water. We now know that Alzheimer's disease can be prevented. However, we will only begin to do so when its primary cause is acknowledged.

CHAPTER 15

Building a Case for Aluminum and Breast Cancer

I have written elsewhere in this book about antiperspirants and their contribution to the body burden of aluminum. The specific case of breast cancer involves another personal recollection. About twenty-five years ago, while I was researching the field of antiperspirants and their links to human disease, the name of Philippa Darbre was preeminent, not at the time with respect to aluminum, but in linking the incidence of breast cancer to the use of antiperspirant. Philippa, an oncologist at Reading University in the United Kingdom, was primarily concerned with a possible role for the preservative parabens in breast cancer. Parabens were commonly added to cosmetics to act as preservatives, and their known estrogenic properties alerted Philippa to the possibility that they might have a role in breast cancer.[1] I contacted Philippa by email, early in the 2000s, and made the suggestion that since the main ingredient in antiperspirants was aluminum, it might also be important in breast cancer. Philippa visited me at Keele soon after, and we forged a long-standing collaboration and, equally important, friendship. It was not long thereafter that Philippa reported in 2005, at the Sixth Keele Meeting on Aluminum in Buçaco, Portugal, that aluminum acted as a metallo-eostrogen, thereby implicating it as an etiological factor in breast cancer. Philippa's assertions were supported by research elsewhere, for example, by Kris McGrath

---

1 Philippa D. Darbre, "Endocrine Disruptors and Obesity," *Current Obesity Reports* 6 (February 15, 2017): 18–27, https://link.springer.com/article/10.1007/s13679-017-0240-4.

in the United States,[2] and it was at this point that we carried out our study into the aluminum content of breast tissue in individuals with breast cancer. The results were intriguing in that, in all tissue donors, we identified a clear regional distribution of aluminum in breast tissue with the outer region (closest to the underarm) having a higher content of aluminum than the inner region.[3] The amount of aluminum in breast tissue varied considerably among tissue donors, but the highest concentrations for each individual were always in tissue adjacent to the underarm. Of course, we speculated that this was due to the application of aluminum-based antiperspirant in the underarm region, though we did not have any direct evidence linked to tissue donors to support such an assertion. In truth, we did not know if donors were regular users of antiperspirants. The charity supporting the tissue donations, the Genesis Appeal, along with their collaborating oncologist, Lester Barr, were somewhat sensitive to the results we obtained and played any media requests to discuss the data with, to use a cricketing term, a dead bat. In other words, they always looked to downplay any suggestion that there might be a link with exposure to aluminum. Something you become accustomed to in aluminum research.

Data on the aluminum content of breast tissue are complicated by the observation that when tissues are dried at 37°C to a constant weight as part of their preparation for subsequent analysis, the breast fat separates from the tissue as a clear oil. I presume that this oil is the form that breast fat takes in the living body. As a quick aside, I worked with one particular female breast cancer oncologist from Austria who refused to acknowledge that her breasts were oil-filled! In our first aforementioned study, we measured the aluminum content of tissue and oil, separately, and the data showing the regional distribution of aluminum across the breast were for tissue, not oil. In a follow-up study, six years later, we measured the aluminum content of whole breast tissue, tissue and oil combined, and did not find a regional distribution of aluminum across the breast.[4] It is observations of this ilk that

2 K G McGrath, "An earlier age of breast cancer diagnosis related to more frequent use of antiperspirants/deodorants and underarm shaving," *Eur J Cancer Prev* 12, no. 6 (December 2003): 479–485, https://pubmed.ncbi.nlm.nih.gov/14639125/.

3 Christopher Exley, Lisa M. Charles, Lester Barr, Claire Martin, Anthony Polwart, and Philippa D. Darbre, "Aluminium in human breast tissue," *Journal of Inorganic Biochemistry* 101, no. 9 (September 2007): 1344–1346, https://www.sciencedirect.com/science/article/pii/S0162013407001304?via%3Dihub.

4 Emily House, Anthony Polwart, Philippa Darbre, Lester Barr, George Metaxas, and Christopher Exley, "The aluminium content of breast tissue taken from women with breast cancer," *Journal of Trace Elements in Medicine and Biology* 27, no. 4 (October 2013): 257–266, https://www.sciencedirect.com/science/article/abs/pii/S0946672X13000576?via%3Dihub.

attest to the difficulties of coming to firm conclusions on a possible role of aluminum in breast cancer, never mind antiperspirants and breast cancer.

However, research from the past five years has changed my thinking from someone who was undecided to someone who now considers a role for aluminum in breast cancer as a very real possibility. The sea change began with an appreciation from published research and our own study that sweating is an important route of excretion of aluminum from the body.[5] Antiperspirants are made of aluminum, usually aluminum chlorohydrate, and could be a source of aluminum in breast tissue. However, antiperspirants are effective because they inhibit the activity of sweat glands, thereby preventing, or at least reducing, sweating. Does this mean that tissues where sweating is inhibited through the application of antiperspirants are predisposed to accumulate more aluminum? Antiperspirants represent the proverbial "double whammy," since they catalyze the accumulation of aluminum in breast tissue both through absorption across the skin from applied product and through prevention of excretion of systemic aluminum in sweat. This new appreciation of the actions of antiperspirants places additional credence upon the results of exceptional animal models of breast cancer, demonstrating that aluminum is a breast carcinogen.[6] The "double-whammy effect" means that there is sufficient time for aluminum to accumulate in breast tissue to a threshold concentration capable of transforming mammary epithelial cells and enabling them to both form tumors and, critically, metastasize. Of course, as with many animal models of human disease, one is reminded that, in this example, mice do not get breast cancer. However, a study out of Innsbruck, Austria, in which I played a small part helped me to conclude that aluminum has a role to play in breast cancer.[7] In an age-matched case control study involving 209 females with breast cancer and 209 healthy controls, it was unequivocally demonstrated that the use of antiperspirants

5 Clare Minshall, Jodie Nadal, and Christopher Exley, "Aluminium in human sweat," *Journal of Trace Elements in Medicine and Biology* 28, no. 1 (January 2014): 87–88, https://www.sciencedirect.com/science/article/abs/pii/S0946672X13001612.

6 Stefano J. Mandriota, Mirna Tenan, Paolo Ferrari, and André-Pascal Sappino, "Aluminium chloride promotes tumorigenesis and metastasis in normal murine mammary gland epithelial cells," *International Journal of Cancer* 139, no. 12 (December 15, 2016): 2781–2790, https://onlinelibrary.wiley.com/doi/full/10.1002/ijc.30393.

7 Caroline Linhart, Heribert Talasz, Evi M. Morandi, Christopher Exley, Herbert H. Lindner, Susanne Taucher, et al., "Use of Underarm Cosmetic Products in Relation to Risk of Breast Cancer: A Case-Control Study," *EBioMedicine* 21 (July 1, 2017): 79–85, https://www.thelancet.com/journals/ebiom/article/PIIS2352-3964(17)30233-5/fulltext.

was significantly associated with risk of breast cancer. The data showed that in women below the age of thirty who used an antiperspirant more than once a day, the risk of breast cancer was four times higher. We—this was my small contribution to the study—also found a significantly higher content of aluminum in defatted breast cancer tissue compared to controls. The latter added further weight to the aforementioned "double-whammy effect" of antiperspirants. The results of this clinical trial were unequivocal about the increased risk of breast cancer in one specific cohort of the tested population. This convinces me that a larger study would extend this risk to all frequent users of antiperspirants. Aluminum should now be considered as the major environmental factor contributing to breast cancer, and its role in the disease is significantly increased through the regular application of aluminum-based antiperspirants.

I have not written specifically about aluminum and cancer in this book. The research on breast cancer, continuing today in the laboratories of inspired individuals like Stefano Mandriota in Geneva, demonstrates that aluminum is a carcinogen. This conclusion is supported by recent science, and I am confident that it will be strengthened by future science. It is of interest to note that science does tend to repeat itself. In the early part of the twentieth century, the Cancer Society of America commissioned a major report on the human health effects of aluminum. This learned society was well aware of the toxicity of the myriad new aluminum products that heralded the advent of the Aluminum Age. It was probably these very real concerns, raised at the beginning of the twentieth century about the toxicity of aluminum in humans that fueled the rise and rise of the all-powerful aluminum industry lobby of today.

CHAPTER 16

Aluminum Is a Genuine Contender as a Cause of Multiple Sclerosis

A serendipitous meeting with Professor Clive Hawkins about fifteen years ago set us on a path toward implicating and understanding a role for aluminum in multiple sclerosis (MS). Clive was professor of Neurology at Keele and an expert in MS. We were initially interested in identifying urinary biomarkers of oxidative damage, the thinking being that the degradation of myelin in MS involved oxidative stress. We (well, my wife, Olga) had developed a method involving reverse phase high performance liquid chromatography (RP HPLC) to identify breakdown products of oxidative damage in human tissues. We used this method to compare the urine of individuals suffering from relaxing remitting (RR) and secondary progressive (SP) MS with that of healthy age and gender-matched controls. In addition to the products of oxidative damage, we also measured in all recruits the urinary excretion of iron and aluminum, both of which are known catalysts of oxidative stress. We could not identify any urinary biomarkers of oxidative stress.

However, what we did find were extraordinarily high concentrations of both iron and aluminum in urine in both RRMS and SPMS compared to controls. We published this research in the journal *Multiple Sclerosis*,[1] and while the data on urinary aluminum excretion in particular were, at the time,

1 Christopher Exley, Godwin Mamutse, Olga Korchazhkina, et al., "Elevated urinary excretion of aluminium and iron in multiple sclerosis," *Multiple Sclerosis Journal* (September 1, 2006) https://journals.sagepub.com/doi/10.1177/1352458506071323.

a surprise, there was a case for saying that we might have expected the results. Why? Well, when I made a closer inspection of the published scientific literature available at the time, it revealed that brain tissue myelin was a consistent target in animal models of aluminum intoxication. Oligodendrocytes, the type of glial cell in the brain responsible for the production of myelin, were shown to be particularly susceptible to the neurotoxicity of aluminum. Indeed, in vitro research also showed that aluminum promoted the oxidative breakdown of myelin. Animal models of intoxication by aluminum were predicting a role for aluminum in MS without invoking such specifically.

Researchers working with these animal models had not made the connection with MS. However, a burgeoning body of research at that time, and indeed up to the present day, links the incidence of autoimmune disease including multiple sclerosis with aluminum adjuvants in vaccines. I have written about these links elsewhere in this book, and they include specific associations with hepatitis B vaccine as well as macrophage myofasciitis (see MMF and Romain Gherardi) and chronic fatigue syndrome. The body of research that suggested a role for aluminum in MS was burgeoning, while research identifying other potential causes of the disease continued to show insignificant progress. While the environment was recognized as being a critical factor in MS, researchers were seemingly going out of their way not to invoke human exposure to aluminum as a possible contributing environmental factor. The stalling and stymying of effective research into an all-too-common neurological condition ring one or two other bells, don't they?, with Alzheimer's disease ringing loudest in my ears.

It took us almost another ten years before we could obtain funding for a follow-up clinical trial to test our observation of a possible role for aluminum in MS.[2] In the new twenty-four-week trial, again with the support of Professor Clive Hawkins, we recruited fifteen individuals diagnosed with progressive MS. For the first twelve weeks of the trial, we collected urine samples so that we could obtain an accurate and long-term record of their urinary excretion of aluminum and with such obtain an estimate of their body burden of aluminum. These data confirmed what we had found in our first clinical trial that individuals with MS, especially females, excrete very high amounts of aluminum in their urine. For the second twelve weeks of

---

2 Krista Jones, Caroline Linhart, Clive Hawkins, and Christopher Exley, "Urinary Excretion of Aluminium and Silicon in Secondary Progressive Multiple Sclerosis," *EBioMedicine* 26 (December 1, 2017): 60–67, https://www.thelancet.com/journals/ebiom/article/PIIS2352-3964(17)30428-0/fulltext.

the trial, we asked the participants to include a silicon-rich mineral water in their daily diets, Spritzer mineral water from Malaysia, and to drink up to 1.5L/day. None of the trial participants found drinking 1.5L/day of Spritzer an onerous task, and compliance was virtually 100 percent for the full twelve weeks. When you drink a silicon-rich mineral water, the silicon content of your urine increases quite significantly, and so it was relatively easy to check if trial recruits had been drinking the water as required.

Analyses of urine samples demonstrated significant increases in the excretion of aluminum for both males and females during the second phase of the trial. These data confirmed what we had observed previously in individuals with Alzheimer's disease and in healthy volunteers—that regular drinking of a silicon-rich mineral water increases the excretion of aluminum from the body in urine. In about half of the participants of the new MS trial, there was evidence from the final week of the trial that the amount of aluminum excreted was diminishing. This observation was interpreted as evidence that in time, regular drinking of silicon-rich mineral waters would lower the body burden of aluminum in individuals with MS. Of course, we never had the opportunity to put that observation to the test. When a clinical trial ends, all involvement with participants in the trial also ends.

However, I say this with one interesting proviso. About one year after the trial had finished and coincidentally almost the same week that the research was published in the journal *EBioMedicine*, I was contacted by email by a local consultant neurologist. They asked if I had carried out a trial in which individuals with MS had been asked to drink mineral water. The neurologist explained that one of their regular patients had participated in the trial and had continued to drink a silicon-rich mineral water each day after the trial had finished. They made the decision to continue, buying a silicon-rich mineral water from their local supermarket, because they had benefited immensely from being part of the trial, and, according to the neurologist, their MS was no longer progressing. I sent the curious neurologist a copy of the hot-off-the-press paper and . . . I never heard from them again! I can only assume that one of the many arms of the aluminum mafia quickly curtailed their innocent interest in our research.

Our observation confirming that individuals with MS have an unusually high body burden of aluminum prompted us to ask the question if some of this aluminum was in brain tissue. If aluminum was contributing to degradation of myelin in MS, then it made sense that we would find aluminum in MS brain tissue. The answer was an unequivocal yes. We measured aluminum in brain tissue from fourteen donors with MS, and all had what we have described as a pathologically significant concentration of aluminum in at least one area of the brain.[3] When the aluminum content of brain tissue in MS was compared with two different control groups, in both cases the elevated levels in MS were highly significant.[4] There can be no doubt that individuals with MS have too much aluminum in their brain tissue and human exposure to aluminum is a likely environmental contributor to the incidence and etiology of MS.[5] In addition to our quantitative analyses, we also used aluminum-specific fluorescence microscopy to identify aluminum in both extracellular and intracellular locations in gray and white matter in MS brain tissue. Aluminum was frequently observed in glial cells, perhaps reflecting the inflammatory nature of MS, and appeared in extracellular structures known as corpora amylacea. The latter are sometimes considered as tombstones of cell death in MS, perhaps similar to senile plaques in Alzheimer's disease and Lewy bodies in Parkinson's disease.

Now that we know that aluminum is a putative causal factor in MS, it is not too difficult to make a link with disease etiology. We know from animal models that aluminum preferentially associates with myelin in brain tissue. Aluminum is a powerful adjuvant. Could its association with myelin catalyze the raising of antibodies against myelin or myelin complexed with aluminum? We know that this is the nature of autoimmunity seen in MS, and I have not read many better explanations of why the body begins to attack and destroy its own myelin. The additional property of aluminum as a very powerful prooxidant[6] would contribute significantly to the degradation of myelin, and this, of course, is where we started our research on MS. We were looking for products of oxidative damage in the urine of MS sufferers.

3 Matthew Mold, Agata Chmielecka, Maria Raquel Ramirez Rodriguez, Femia Thom, Caroline Linhart, Andrew King, and Christopher Exley, "Aluminium in Brain Tissue in Multiple Sclerosis," *International Journal of Environmental Research and Public Health* 15, no. 8 (August 18, 2018): 1777, https://www.mdpi.com/1660-4601/15/8/1777.

4 C. Linhart, D. Davidson, S. Pathmanathan, T. Kamaladas, and C. Exley, "Aluminium in Brain Tissue in Non-neurodegenerative/Non-neurodevelopmental Disease: A Comparison with Multiple Sclerosis," *Exposure and Health* (February 25, 2020) https://link.springer.com /article/10.1007%2Fs12403-020-00346-9.

5 Christopher Exley and Elizabeth Clarkson, "Aluminium in human brain tissue from donors without neurodegenerative disease: A comparison with Alzheimer's disease, multiple sclerosis and autism," *Scientific Reports* 10 (May 8, 2020), https://www.nature.com/articles/s41598 -020-64734-6.

6 Christopher Exley, "The pro-oxidant activity of aluminum," *Free Radical Biology and Medicine* 36, no. 3 (Ferbraury 2004): 380–387, https://www.sciencedirect.com/science/article/abs/pii /S0891584903007937?via%3Dihub.

CHAPTER 17

A Top Trumps Mechanism of Aluminum Toxicity

A long conversation could be had unraveling the complexities behind what makes something toxic. Toxicity is a major force propelling Darwinian natural selection. For example, it is why we breathe oxygen and why we use calcium to make an endoskeleton. Toxicity is a change in the status quo and presents a challenge to all exposed biota. It works at the cellular, tissue, and whole organism level. The latter reminds me of a recent question at home concerning why only dwarf varieties of a certain thistle thrive in my field. The answer lies in the toxicity exerted by a lawn mower every second week. Only those plants whose genetic makeup supports rapid growth to flower and seed thrive in grass cut every two weeks. This is Darwinian natural selection in action and not Lamarckism, thistles "learning" to adapt to their new surroundings!

All biota, including my thistles, are composed of populations of individuals differing by myriad mutations in their genome, and it is the nature of these differences in any specific environment that determines which prosper. My dwarf thistles are identical species to my tall thistles. The former have a different genetic makeup that gives them the advantage in the environment of a cut lawn. In my adjacent wildflower field, where the grass is not cut, mainly tall thistles are found. Being short in tall grass is not an advantage for this thistle.

Aluminum is toxic because it disrupts cellular biochemistry. This is why it kills fish in acid waters and destroys trees in catchments affected by acid rain. It is also why renal patients died of dialysis encephalopathy. The problem in defining why, or perhaps how, aluminum is toxic lies in deciding which cellular biochemistry is most affected in which environment. The latter, the physicochemical compartment housing the biochemistry, is perhaps most critical. The relatively small size and comparatively large charge of biologically reactive aluminum, $Al^{3+}_{(aq)}$ make it an ideal metal-cofactor for oxygen-based functional groups on myriad biomolecules. Fluoride functional groups also bind aluminum with high avidity, especially in slightly acidic compartments.

I recently had an illuminating if also mildly bizarre discussion with a small group of highly esteemed scientists, including a chemistry Nobel laureate, at a university in California. The discussion, originally relating to the putative toxicity of glyphosate in humans, raised the somewhat alarming suggestion, apparently coming from the chemistry laureate, that the spike proteins on COVID-19 were fluoridated. I was forced to point out that since there were no naturally occurring fluoridated proteins, this was unlikely or, alternatively, this would prove that COVID-19 was man-made. The prospect of a nonstick "Teflon" virus intrigued me. Nonetheless, the discussion went quiet after this, but it did set me thinking about the potential repercussions of fluoridated ligands for the toxicity of aluminum and specifically implications for the widespread and continuous prescription of fluoroquinolone antibiotics. However, for now in considering aluminum's toxicity, we can restrict thinking to oxygen-based functional groups, and there are plenty of these. If we allow for a ready and infinite supply of biologically reactive aluminum, then an array of ligands will compete to bind aluminum. These ligands could include pyrophosphate groups on nucleotides like ATP, carboxylic acid groups on organic acids such as citrate, and infinite combinations of hydroxyl, carbonyl, phosphate, and carboxylic acid groups on proteins and amino acids, the latter including neurotransmitters such as glutamate. The binding of aluminum by each group or combination of groups is the first step in an equilibrium, and together competitive equilibria involving aluminum and all these possible groups define the fate of aluminum and any subsequent possible toxicity.

To understand this further, we need to go back to Darwinian natural selection, especially the concept of "survival of the fittest." This is often wrongly interpreted as biggest, strongest, fastest, etc., is best and ultimately the winner. However, the critical term is "fittest," and this brings the environment to the fore. For example, in the highly competitive world of ligands binding biologically reactive aluminum, small changes in the environment housing the biochemistry have significant impact upon which of the competitive equilibria triumphs. In its simplest form, a change in pH from 5.5 to 6.0 switches the triumphant ligand from fluoride to hydroxyl and is hence why the former increases the absorption of aluminum across the stomach but not the latter regions of the small intestine. Another very important factor is the relative concentrations of ligands competing to bind aluminum. Imagine, as I do, and paint a picture in your head. Each competitive ligand binds aluminum, and the resulting chemical bond has a finite lifetime. Aluminum remains bound for a specific time. There is an aluminum on and an aluminum off state. When the ligand concentration is relatively high, the on rate is favored. In a dilute environment, the off rate is favored, and such circumstances offer opportunities for competing ligands to steal aluminum, thereby forming a different complex. Depending upon the environment where biologically reactive aluminum is present, any number of potential ligands compete to bind and retain aluminum. If binding aluminum, perhaps in preference to the evolutionarily selected metal cofactor, disrupts the function or role of the winning biomolecule, then toxicity ensues. The acuity of any resulting toxicity depends upon the extent to which the affected system is disrupted and whether or not there are any compensatory systems immediately accessible.

There are myriad such opportunities for aluminum toxicity in the human body. However, what might be the Top Trumps mechanism whereby aluminum exerts everyday toxicity in the body? I have thought about this often, and I have nearly always concluded that I cannot make this choice. How can I choose between so many potential competitive equilibria? If I am going to be pushed to make a decision on this, then I am going to choose a ligand and its complex with aluminum that, as yet, has only been proven to exist in silico. In 2004, I proposed the existence of the aluminum superoxide semireduced radical ion $AlO_2^{\bullet 2+}$. I suggested that the formation of this complex was behind the unexplained prooxidant property of the non-redox active aluminum in catalyzing both iron and non-iron dependent oxidative damage across biota.[1] While world-class computational chemistry has proven both the existence and prooxidant activity of $AlO_2^{\bullet 2+}$,[2] it remains to be identified directly in any biological milieu. However, oxidative damage

1 Christopher Exley, "The pro-oxidant activity of aluminum," https://www.sciencedirect.com/science/article/abs/pii/S0891584903007937?via%3Dihub.

2 J. I. Mujika, F. Ruipérez, I. Infante, J. M. Ugalde, C. Exley, and X. Lopez, "Pro-oxidant Activity of Aluminum: Stabilization of the Aluminum Superoxide Radical Ion," *Journal of Physical Chemistry* A 115, no. 24 (May 23, 2011): 6717–6723, https://pubs.acs.org/doi/10.1021/jp203290b.

underlies much human disease, including neurodegenerative disease, and its ubiquity equally supports integral roles for aluminum in catalyzing such damage, potentially changing oxidative damage from something that, in the absence of aluminum, is relatively benign to something that is manifested as toxicity. Forced to choose one mechanism of aluminum toxicity as being of greatest significance, I would focus upon the now-explained, prooxidant activity of aluminum. However, we are oxidative metabolizers, and our bodies are replete with essential antioxidants. Indeed, antioxidants are effective in protecting against the prooxidant activity of aluminum.

In order to understand why aluminum-promoted oxidative damage underlies human diseases, especially those associated with the brain, we need to think about redox chemistry in the light of natural selection. We are effective oxidative metabolizers because oxidative biochemistry evolved alongside antioxidant biochemistry. The oxidant and the antioxidant are present within the same biological compartment. Redox toxicity only ensues when these coupled biochemical systems are separated in either space or time, or both. The separation may occur due to a disruption in antioxidant biochemistry, or it may be caused by anomalous oxidative biochemistry. The latter was of interest to us. We investigated why senile plaques in Alzheimer's disease brain tissue were apparent sources, or possibly sinks, of oxidative tissue damage. In an in vitro study, we showed that senile plaques acted as a nidus for redox cycling of iron, iron (III) being reduced to the oxidative damaging iron (II) in a continuous cycle.[3] The presence of aluminum pushed the redox equilibrium significantly in favor of iron (II), thus exacerbating the potential for oxidative damage. Senile plaques were sources of redox active iron (II), and their extracellular location in brain tissue separated this oxidative chemistry from any immediately available antioxidant chemistry. The result was significant tissue—neuronal—damage in the immediate vicinities of these deposits of fibrillary amyloid-β. Of significant interest was that the presence of copper (II) in the senile plaque structures acted as an antioxidant pushing the redox cycle back toward iron (III). We actually found good evidence for protective effects of copper (II) in our study on aluminum, iron, copper, and amyloid-β in sporadic Alzheimer's disease.[4]

3 Ayesha Khan, Jon P. Dobson, and Christopher Exley, "Redox cycling of iron by Aβ42," *Free Radical Biology and Medicine* 40, no. 4 (February 15, 2006): 557–569, https://www.sciencedirect.com/science/article/abs/pii/S0891584905005332?via%3Dihub.

4 Christopher Exley, Emily House, Anthony Polwart, and Margaret M. Esiri, "Brain Burdens of Aluminum, Iron, and Copper and their Relationships with Amyloid-β Pathology in 60 Human Brains," *Journal of Alzheimer's Disease* 31, no. 4 (September 11, 2012): 725–730, https://content.iospress.com/articles/journal-of-alzheimers-disease/jad120766.

What I have termed anomalous or unexpected prooxidative biochemistry, iron-dependent or otherwise, will be significantly accelerated by the additional presence of aluminum acting through $AlO_2\bullet^{2+}$, and this is why I have chosen the prooxidant activity of aluminum as my "Top Trumps" of mechanisms of aluminum toxicity. I have been asked many times if aluminum might exert its toxicity by a particular mechanism, and my usual answer is yes, that is possible and I might even add that such a mechanism of action has been demonstrated in vitro, in cell models, and in animal models. Understanding the toxicity of aluminum in humans is less about the identification of a specific mechanism, since there are myriad potential mechanisms, and much more about the probability that biologically reactive aluminum will be in the right place at the right time in sufficient quantity to manifest toxicity in the body. Aluminum is only toxic; it really should not be in the body.

CHAPTER 18

Camelford—Anatomy of a Government Cover-up

Camelford is a small Cornish town made infamous as the center of the United Kingdom's worst-known mass poisoning of the human population. On July 6, 1988, twenty tons of aluminum sulphate, routinely used throughout the country in the treatment of potable water, was added by mistake directly into treated water supplying twenty thousand people in Camelford and surrounding areas. At that time in the United Kingdom, the supply of clean drinking water was under public ownership, but it was about to be privatized in a share offer to the public. This reference to the eventual privatization of potable water supplies throughout England and Wales in 1989 is of significance, as it is widely accepted to be the basis of the cover-up that followed and continues to this day.

While I had remained in touch with everything that followed the incident in 1988, my personal involvement with Camelford began much later with the opening of a new inquiry in 2001 by the then-Labor Environment Minister, Michael Meacher. He announced adamantly that "all the health consequences of the incident would be uncovered." However, upon perusing the details available concerning the new inquiry, I immediately smelled the proverbial rat. The experts appointed to the Department of Health, Committee on Toxicology (DH COT), to review Camelford had absolutely no relevant (or even irrelevant) expertise in aluminum, health-related or otherwise. They were simply a hotchpotch of individuals drafted in, presumably, from other DH COT panels. The only legitimate appointees to the expert panel were probably the two lay members representing the citizens of Camelford, Doug Cross and Peter Smith.

As an independent university-funded scientist who, in 2001, had a burgeoning reputation for research on aluminum and human health (for example, I had just edited an acclaimed book on aluminum and Alzheimer's disease),[1] I waited in vain to be called to give evidence to the expert panel. Instead, somewhat frustrated, I made contact with them and specifically a member of the secretariat, George Kowalczyk. George was actually enthusiastic to receive my input and almost immediately asked me to write a report detailing aluminum chemistry and toxicology relevant to Camelford. I was then asked to give evidence to the expert panel in person and answer questions on my report. Upon doing so, the committee chair, Professor Frank Woods, went out of his way to thank me personally and asked if I would be prepared to help the committee in drafting the section of their report that covered the environmental toxicology of aluminum. Of course, I agreed, and I left the DH COT meeting in London with a degree of optimism that something might actually be done about Camelford. I never heard from Frank Woods again with respect to this request. Even esteemed chairs of government committees can be nobbled!

When eventually the DH COT draft report was published in 2005, it did not contain any of the information I had provided as written or oral evidence. It was clear from the draft report that another government cover-up was in the making. To all intents and purposes, aluminum, in particular, would not be considered as a critical criterion in their investigation of Camelford including, to quote Michael Meacher, all the consequences for the health of the affected population. Twenty thousand people had been poisoned by drinking tap water containing 600 mg/L aluminum over a period of several weeks, and the committee charged with investigating the disaster was not considering any possible ill effects relating to exposure to aluminum. The so-called expert committee was certainly not interested in delving into the science that supported aluminum as the key contaminant in this event. I wrote a letter to the British Medical Journal to this effect. The letter was cosigned by more than fifty aluminum scientists from around the

---

1 *Aluminium and Alzheimer's Disease: The Science that Describes the Link*, ed. Christopher Exley (Elsevier Science, 2001), https://www.sciencedirect.com/book/9780444508119/aluminium -and-alzheimers-disease.

world.[2] I have copied this letter below just in case it becomes unavailable through the *BMJ*:

Aluminum and Camelford

In 2001, the enquiry into the contamination by aluminum sulphate of the public water supply of a large area of North Cornwall, centred around the town of Camelford, was re-opened. An independent expert advisory committee, the Committee on Toxicity of Chemicals in Food, Consumer Products and the Environment (COT) were asked by the Department of Health (DH) to advise on whether the pollution incident had resulted in delayed or persistent health effects and on the need for additional monitoring and research. COT have now made available for consultation the draft report of their investigation. We have a number of general criticisms concerning the way in which COT have dealt with issues concerning the exposure of the local population to the known environmental toxin, aluminum.

(i) The subgroup appointed to the enquiry did not include anyone with any direct experience of any aspect of the chemistry or environmental toxicology of aluminum. We asked at the outset that this shortcoming should be rectified but the request went unheeded and it is now clear that this mistake has resulted in an entirely inadequate treatment of the role played by aluminum in this incident. It is not the purpose of this letter to review the many ways in which the report has failed in its consideration of any role played by aluminum, this will be done in full as part of the so-called consultation process, but as a background to these misgivings it may suffice to point out that the subgroup's report makes reference to only six (6) peer-reviewed publications on aluminum since 2001, a period in which in excess of 350 papers of potential relevance to the enquiry were published (data easily available via ISI Web of Science). One of these six publications, Priest (2004), is repeatedly referenced and is written by an individual who gave oral evidence to the subgroup on behalf of the Aluminum Federation!

(ii) The great majority of the water quality data used by the subgroup in arriving at their conclusions was provided by the South West Water Authority (SWWA). Regardless of the fact that independent analyses were

---

2 Christopher Exley et al., "Inquiry questions long term effects on health of Camelford incident," *BMJ* 330 (February 3, 2005) https://www.bmj.com/rapid-response/2011/10/30/aluminium -and-camelford.

only scarcely available (though some that were came from the Laboratory of the Government Chemist at Taunton) it is surprising that the subgroup have chosen to use data provided by the 'polluters'. These data have not been critically appraised by the subgroup. We are not offered any information about the methods which were used to determine aluminum in the water samples. It is notoriously difficult to measure high concentrations of aluminum (> mg/L) with any degree of confidence and there is evidence from the data provided by SWWA that their measurements for aluminum are significantly lower than would have been predicted from the corresponding concentrations of sulphate. Intriguingly these disparities between the aluminum and sulphate concentrations are only evident for those water samples taken at the outset of the incident when the corresponding concentrations of aluminum in the water supplies would have been expected to have been at their highest.

(iii)   We do not wish to argue with the recommendations for further research. These ostensibly amount to every area in which aluminum exposure might impact upon human health and are to be applauded. The surprise is that considering these recommendations the subgroup were still able to conclude that 'it is not anticipated that the increased exposure to aluminum would have caused, or would be expected to cause, delayed or persistent harm to those who were adults or toddlers at the time of the incident'. It is difficult to reconcile the recommendations for further research with the unequivocal nature of the conclusion on human health.

It is our contention that the conclusions drawn by the subgroup concerning aluminum have been drawn from an entirely inadequate data base both with respect to the literature that has been reviewed and cited in the report and the water quality analyses provided by SWWA. In relation to the former, it would have been welcomed if the subgroup had pointed out that the United Kingdom government through for example, the research councils etc. have not funded any independent research on aluminum and health in the last decade, if not longer, and that this inexplicable breakdown in research funding might have contributed to their difficulties in reviewing the toxicological consequences of the poisoning of the Camelford public water supply by aluminum. Fortunately, first class research from outside of the United Kingdom has ensured that we are much better informed than the subgroup has demonstrated in its review of the literature. We do not think that the proposed period of consultation (up to the 22nd April 2005) will be sufficient neither to remedy the deficiencies of this report nor to do justice to the concerns of the people affected by this incident.

Christopher Exley PhD (and 50 further signatories.)

Considering the clear inadequacies of the report, one has to ask the question as to what changed Frank Woods's mind about his suggestion of having me draft the part of the report concerning the environmental toxicology of aluminum. How and by whom was he nobbled? Could it have had anything to do with the fact that the day after he asked for my help his committee took evidence from two individuals, Nick Priest and James Edwardson, on behalf of the Aluminum Federation?[3] I was told by the Department of Health's representative on the inquiry, Frances Pollitt, that it was a complete coincidence that these two well-known "aluminum ambassadors" (my name for the army of so-called scientists paid by the aluminum industry to dispute all health effects attributable to aluminum) gave their evidence the day after me. I was also informed that they, like me, had offered to give evidence to the inquiry and had not been asked to give evidence. It is, I am sure you can agree, quite a coincidence in an inquiry period stretching over several years that these aluminum ambassadors not only offered to give evidence at much the same time as myself, but also were asked to do so immediately following my evidence. However, I asked if it was also a complete coincidence that, just a few years earlier in 1999, the aforementioned Frances Pollitt had been the individual at the Department of Health who had signed off a grant for £100,000 to the Aluminum Federation's Nick Priest to carry out research on aluminum and human health. I think that we can all surmise that once George Kowalczyk had informed the committee, and therefore Pollitt, that I would be giving evidence, Pollitt was immediately in touch with Priest to solicit their offer of evidence. Pollitt acted as a conduit between the aluminum industry and government, and her actions in this respect were to become even more obvious, as the fallout from Camelford began to involve more and more affected Camelford families. Going back to her connections with Priest (see Priest speaking in Bert Ehgartner's seminal documentary *The Aluminum Files*[4] to get a flavor of his colors), it is somewhat ironic, if also absurd, that the only grant (probably ever) to research aluminum and human health awarded directly by the British Government was to a consultant to the aluminum industry.

The consultancy was a fact that Priest was completely open about in his grant application document. The £100K grant accepted and spent by Priest subsequently never produced a single published outcome. The last time that I wrote to the Department of Health to inquire about this, I was told that they were still waiting for the final report on the project. This was in 2006.

---

3 Aluminum Federation home page, accessed October 1, 2020, https://alfed.org.uk/.
4 "The Age of Aluminium (Die Akte Aluminium)," accessed October 1, 2020, https://www .youtube.com/watch?v=5F0u54gs0iU&t=120s.

This is just one further aspect of the scandal, that British taxpayers were not only poisoned by Camelford, but also contributed financially to its cover up by the government. I am sure that Pollitt was charged by the government to get the DH COT draft report on Camelford accepted and published as soon as possible so as to draw a line under Camelford once and for all. But neither Ms. Pollitt nor the government was prepared for what happened next!

I met Doug Cross for the first time in 1999, if I remember correctly, at an Environmental Assistance conference in Northern Ireland where I was talking, unsurprisingly, about the environmental toxicology of aluminum. Doug introduced himself as a forensic ecologist, and, in truth, I did not really understand what that meant and I do not remember much else about our personal meeting. The next time we met was a few years later, when I gave my evidence to the DH COT expert panel on Camelford. While Doug was on the panel as a so-called lay member, it was immediately obvious that he knew substantially more about aluminum as an environmental toxin than any of the "experts." He asked inquisitive and, at times, incisive questions, and it was clear that he wanted to know and understand the role played by aluminum in the incident. After this meeting, Doug stayed in touch with me through the occasional email. What happened next must go down in the annals of serendipity. Perhaps not with respect to Doug Cross, as you will shortly read, but in the whole and sorry affair that is Camelford.

Shortly after the release in 2005 of the DH COT Draft Report on Camelford, I received a telephone call from Doug. He was to the point. He told me that his wife had died, that the circumstances of her death were unusual, and that he wanted me to organize a postmortem on his wife's brain. That was an unusual telephone conversation, as you can imagine. Doug's wife was forty-four when she, like many, was exposed to high levels of aluminum in Camelford drinking water. Fifteen years later in May 2003, she was experiencing poor mental health, and, in April 2004, she died. Because of the unusual circumstances and a lack of consensus among health practitioners as to the cause of her death, the Taunton coroner, Michael Rose, agreed to further analyses of her brain tissue.

Following on from Doug's personal request, I asked one of the world's leading neuropathologists at that time, Professor Margaret Esiri at Oxford University, if she would carry out the detailed neuropathology required, and she agreed. Professor Esiri found that Doug's wife had died of an aggressive form of Alzheimer's disease characterized by extensive congophilic amyloid angiopathy (CAA). Professor Esiri noted that the detail of the case was probably unique and certainly so for someone in their fifties. The coroner raised the question of aluminum and Camelford, and Professor Esiri organized for me to receive five samples of cortical brain tissue, the Camelford case and four others from donors to the Oxford Brain Bank. We measured the aluminum content of the tissues blind, and only one gave a high value for aluminum, actually a *very* high concentration of aluminum. It was the Camelford case, and four further brain tissue samples from Doug's wife's brain confirmed the high content of aluminum in this case.

As might be imagined, a small earthquake of interest in Camelford ensued, fueled by significant media interest. In those dim and distant days, the press and associated media were still allowed to report upon the toxicity of aluminum in humans. The subject was not taboo as it is today. Professor Esiri and I, with consent from Doug and the coroner, decided to write up the results as a case report for publication in a medical journal. While *The Lancet* shied away from reviewing the manuscript, in spite of a telephone conversation that had encouraged its submission, the *Journal of Neurology, Neurosurgery and Psychiatry* reviewed and accepted the manuscript within just a few weeks. The scientific paper that followed in early 2006 was titled "Severe cerebral congophilic angiopathy coincident with increased brain aluminum in a resident of Camelford, Cornwall, UK," and its impact was that the DH COT Draft Report was to remain a draft report for another eight years.[5] There are times in science, as in life, when serendipity simply takes over the course of events. The coroner opened an inquest into the death of Doug's wife, and he, unlike the aforementioned promise on Camelford by Michael Meacher MP, would leave no stone unturned in finding the truth behind her death. Part of the inquest involved his asking Somerset County Council to fund what became our seminal study on the aluminum content of sixty human brains.[6] Without this funding, which amounted to over £100,000, it would not have been possible to know everything that we know today concerning aluminum in human brain tissue. If the coroner's inquiry into the death of Carole Cross achieved nothing else, the opportunity to carry out our sixty human brain study was a landmark moment in our research and research generally on aluminum in human neurological

---

5 C Exley and M M Esiri, "Severe cerebral congophilic angiopathy coincident with increased brain aluminium in a resident of Camelford, Cornwall, UK," *Journal of Neurology, Neurosurgery and Psychiatry* 77, no. 7 (2006): 877–879, https://jnnp.bmj.com/content/77/7/877.

6 House, Esiri, Forster, Ince, and Exley, "Aluminium, iron and copper in human brain tissues donated to the medical research council's cognitive function and ageing study," *Metallomics*, https://pubs.rsc.org/en/content/articlelanding/2012/MT/C1MT00139F#!divAbstract.

disease. It has been a catalyst for change and one that now sees aluminum in brain tissue at the proverbial heart of a number of neurodegenerative diseases. We now know that aluminum plays a part in Alzheimer's disease and almost certainly has a role in multiple sclerosis, autism, and Parkinson's disease, too.

Of course, the inquest achieved a great deal, and it was an unusual experience giving evidence in a coroner's court in the spring of 2012. The courtroom in Taunton was traditional and foreboding, the latter accentuated on the day I attended by the presence of several men in dark suits who sat and listened but communicated with no one, neither with themselves nor with the government's representatives of the now- and then-privatized water industry. Following several days of deliberations and hearing evidence, the coroner delivered a narrative verdict, but in so doing, he made it very clear that all of the evidence pointed toward a role for aluminum in the death of Mrs. Cross. It was a narrative verdict because it was impossible to link the aluminum in her brain tissue directly with Camelford. I am sure that this verdict came as some relief to the government and, indeed, to the men in dark suits. However, it set a very important precedent. It is the first, and to my knowledge last, time that in a court of law aluminum was found guilty of causing Alzheimer's disease. The coroner, a very good man, was ahead of his time since it was several years later in 2017 before I was prepared to unequivocally convict aluminum of the same crime.[7]

About a year after the inquest, in 2013, the final DH COT report on Camelford was published.[8] It included only minor concessions to the case of Mrs. Cross, and these were worded in the form of suggestions for future research. The cover-up was now complete, and the "expert panel" dissolved in the becalmed Camelford waters. A number of meetings involving the DH COT Chair Frank Woods, Frances Pollitt, Margaret Esiri, and I followed. However, these were sullied by the presence of a representative from the aluminum industry, Professor Carol Brayne, a Cambridge epidemiologist working on Alzheimer's disease. No explanation was offered for her involvement in the postreport discussions, though the fact, as it transpired, that she headed the study that supplied us with brains for our seminal sixty

7 Exley, "Aluminum Should Now Be Considered a Primary Etiological Factor in Alzheimer's Disease," *Journal of Alzheimer's Disease Reports*, https://content.iospress.com/articles/journal -of-alzheimers-disease-reports/adr170010.

8 Committee on Toxicity of Chemicals in Food, Consumer Products and the Environment, "SUBGROUP REPORT ON THE LOWERMOOR WATER POLLUTION INCIDENT," February 2013, https://cot.food.gov.uk/sites/default/files/cot/lwpiapp811.pdf.

brain study may have been a factor. Brayne showed her true aluminum colors when, upon the completion of our blind measurements of aluminum in brain tissue, she retroactively prevented us from knowing the clinical status of the sixty donor brains. Up until this point in time, she had had no involvement in our request for brain tissues or any other aspect of the following research. Now she insisted that only her research team should carry out statistical analyses of the data from the donor brains.

Of course, we were not prepared to hand over our unpublished data to a representative of the aluminum industry. Individuals such as Brayne, Priest, and Edwardson masquerade as legitimate scientists, while acting to suppress science on behalf of hidden paymasters. We published our sixty human brain data in two separate papers,[9] and Brayne, continuing to the last, even roped in the chair of the brain bank, Dame Ingrid Allen, to write to both the vice-chancellor at Keele, Professor Nick Foskett, and the editor-in-chief of one of the journals, Professor George Perry, to try to prevent publication of the data. I am happy to say that, in this instance at least, academic freedom and transparency of information prevailed, and Brayne's efforts were in vain.[10] Readers will not be surprised to learn that the recommendations for further research made in the Camelford Final Report in 2013 have been totally ignored. However, we have had the opportunity through coroners' and family requests to investigate brain tissue from three individuals known to have been affected by Camelford. In each case, we have found elevated levels of aluminum coincident with unusual neuropathology directly linked to (i) congophilic amyloid angiopathy[11] (an example of early onset Alzheimer's disease),[12] (ii) sporadic or

9 House, Esiri, Forster, Ince, and Exley, "Aluminium, iron and copper in human brain tissues donated to the medical research council's cognitive function and ageing study," *Metallomics*, https://pubs.rsc.org/en/content/articlelanding/2012/MT/C1MT00139F#!divAbstract.

10 Exley, House, Polwart, and Esiri, "Brain Burdens of Aluminum, Iron, and Copper and their Relationships with Amyloid-β Pathology in 60 Human Brains," *Journal of Alzheimer's Disease*, https://content.iospress.com/articles/journal-of-alzheimers-disease/jad120766.

11 Matthew Mold, Jason Cottle, Andrew King, and Christopher Exley, "Intracellular Aluminium in Inflammatory and Glial Cells in Cerebral Amyloid Angiopathy: A Case Report," *Int. J. Environ. Res. Public Health* 16, no. 8 (April 24, 2019): 1459 https://www.mdpi.com/1660-4601/16/8/1459.

12 A. King, C. Troakes, M. Aizpurua, A. Mirza, A. Hodges, S. Al-Sarraj, and C. Exley, "Unusual neuropathological features and increased brain aluminium in a resident of Camelford, UK," *Neuropathology and Applied Neurobiology* 43, no. 6 (October 2017): 537–541, https://onlinelibrary.wiley.com/doi/full/10.1111/nan.12417.

late onset Alzheimer's disease,[13] and (iii) adult onset epilepsy.[14] Three out of three cases implicate aluminum in disease etiology. One is left wondering what might have been found if there had not been a cover-up. Of course, the cover-up also prevented any therapeutic interventions, and we cannot know how much suffering and loss of life might have been avoided if the serious nature of this event had been openly acknowledged from the outset.[15]

13   Mirza, King, Troakes, and Exley, "The Identification of Aluminum in Human Brain Tissue Using Lumogallion and Fluorescence Microscopy," *Journal of Alzheimer's Disease*, https://content .iospress.com/articles/journal-of-alzheimers-disease/jad160648.

14   Matthew Mold, Jason Cottle, and Christopher Exley, "Aluminium in Brain Tissue in Epilepsy: A Case Report from Camelford," *Int. J. Environ. Res. Public Health* 16, no. 12 (June 16, 2019): 2129, https://www.mdpi.com/1660-4601/16/12/2129.

15   Professor Chris Exley, "Camelford: Britain's Forgotten Aluminium Scandal," *The Hippocratic Post*, April 29, 2019, https://www.hippocraticpost.com/neurology/camelford-britains-forgotten-aluminium-scandal/.

CHAPTER 19

Politics

I can still recall a period of blissful naivety in my life of aluminum research. Over thirty years ago when I discovered, as part of my PhD research, that silicon protected against the toxicity of aluminum, my scientific mentor, the late, great polymath JD Birchall OBE FRS, said to me that the results should be written up and submitted as soon as possible to the journal *Nature*. This, submitting to *Nature*, now thought of as the world's leading science journal, meant nothing to me at the time, and since I was busy writing up my thesis, I invited him to write and submit the manuscript. The subject of acid rain and fish deaths was, for want of a better word, fashionable at the time, and the manuscript was submitted and accepted for publication within just a few weeks. Remember that what we now call the Internet was a nascent tool at this time in the late 1980s, and so peer review of manuscripts through the Royal Mail postal system was usually a long and drawn-out affair. Speaking of drawing, figures for the paper were drawn by hand on tracing paper back then. That seminal paper was my first and only publication in *Nature*.[1] It certainly made a useful addendum to my PhD thesis, and, on the occasion of my PhD viva, it clearly impressed my external examiner, the ecotoxicologist Frank Moriarty.

However, the fickle nature of scientific publishing meant that within just a couple of years, the subject of aluminum as the ubiquitous ecotoxin

---

1 J. D. Birchall, C. Exley, J. S. Chappell, and M. J. Phillips, "Acute toxicity of aluminium to fish eliminated in silicon-rich acid waters," *Nature* 338 (March 9, 1989): 146–148, https://www.nature.com/articles/338146a0.

was no longer de rigueur, and aluminum and human health specifically was quickly to become a taboo subject. Academic journals such as *Nature* are wholly reliant upon their sponsors and advertisements, and, regardless of their myriad disclaimers to this effect, these influences clearly dictate what their fresh-faced editorial teams deem as being of interest to their readers. Just compare the type and number of advertisements in a hard copy of *Nature* in 1989 to today in 2020. You will quickly understand who is pulling the strings of scientific freedom at this world-renowned journal. There was a time when I continued naively to submit our best science to *Nature* and other self-proclaimed high-esteem journals. However, our manuscripts submitted to *Nature, Science,* et al. were never peer-reviewed by these journals; they never got past the journals' editorial Mafiosi. This increasing tendency by editorial staff to choose to review subject matter and not science becomes very time-consuming for the submitting scientist and might involve rewriting a manuscript several times before finding a journal that will send it for peer review. I no longer participate in this charade and now only submit our science to an appropriate journal where I can be sure that it will be peer-reviewed. Of course, the latter is also fraught with individual politics and beliefs; you will not be surprised to learn that many so-called peers also only review the subject of a manuscript and not the science therein. But at least it is peer-reviewed, and there is an opportunity to defend your science and its importance.

Disciples of the aluminum industry have infiltrated all of the mechanisms underlying the basic processes of doing science. They sit on grant-giving bodies and they influence what research is published and where. While there is scant if any evidence that the aluminum industry funds independent basic research into aluminum and its effects in biota, their influence upon the subject is far from benign. For example, to the naive scientist researching aluminum for the first time, it may seem that the aluminum industry is contributing toward knowledge on the subject through the publication, every ten years or so, of seemingly authoritative reviews. However, we are being deceived. These are divisive practices, and the publications are designed to act as smokescreens, distractions from the underlying devastation caused by biologically available aluminum. I will recall one classic example of such a practice now.

In 2007, a paper appeared in the *Journal of Toxicology and Environmental Health* (JTEH) purporting to review the risk to human health of aluminum.[2] On the surface, it appeared to originate from an academic department in Canada and included in the list of coauthors one or two with a background in aluminum and human health. One of the coauthors of the paper was the editor-in-chief of JTEH, Sam Kacew. One might wonder why he was a coauthor having no previous background in the subject of aluminum and human health. The answer to this seeming conundrum will soon become obvious to you. While I had known about the existence of this so-called review from a longtime colleague, Bob Yokel, one of the coauthors, I first saw a copy of the accepted manuscript in August 2007 when I received it as part of a review I was undertaking of another manuscript. It was dated February 13, 2007, and hidden away in the "Acknowledgements" was the suggestion that it had been funded by the International Aluminum Institute.[3] However, no conflict of interests had been declared by any of the coauthors. One might have expected funding from the aluminum industry to be considered a conflict. I made a few discrete inquiries and quickly learned that each author had been paid $1,000 for their contribution. I also ascertained that the manuscript had not undergone any form of anonymous peer review. The latter is the gold standard in academic journal publishing and would certainly be expected of a reputable journal like JTEH. Perhaps most surprising of all was that the manuscript had been accepted for publication by one of its authors, the editor-in-chief of JTEH, Sam Kacew.

When I challenged the editors of JTEH with this information, I did not receive a reply from anyone on the journal's editorial board, and so I passed my grievance on to the publishers, Taylor and Francis (T&F). Initially they were also reluctant to provide any information and simply acknowledged receipt of my correspondence. They only conceded to begin to address the issues I raised after several months. One can only guess that they were spending this time devising their "get out of this mess" strategy. Eventually I received email correspondence in which they agreed that all authors had been paid for their contribution, but, surprisingly, they did not believe that payment supported by the International Aluminum Institute constituted a conflict of interests for the authors. They agreed that the manuscript had not undergone any form of anonymous peer review but again T&F did not

---

2 Daniel Krewski, Robert A Yokel, Evert Nieboer, David Borchelt, Joshua Cohen, Jean Harry, Sam Kacew, Joan Lindsay, Amal M Mahfouz, and Virginie Rondeau, "Human Health Risk Assessment for Aluminium, Aluminium Oxide, and Aluminium Hydroxide," *Journal of Toxicology and Environmental Health* 10 (April 7, 2007): 1–269, https://www.tandfonline.com/doi/abs/10.1080/10937400701597766.

3 World Aluminum home page, accessed October 1, 2020, http://www.world-aluminium.org/.

see that this posed a problem. They confirmed with me that Editor-in-Chief Sam Kacew, who was also one of the paid contributors to the review, had accepted the manuscript for publication on behalf of *JTEH*. T&F informed me that they viewed this as simply a formality, though they admitted that it should not happen again in the future, and they asked me, somewhat sheepishly, how I knew about this. I knew because one of the coauthors had sent me a copy of the signed acceptance letter for the manuscript.

The publishers did not take my complaint any further except to include an amended Disclaimer/Acknowledgements statement in the final published version of the paper. Despite the acknowledgement by T&F that all authors, including the editor-in-chief of *JTEH*, were paid for their contribution and that the International Aluminum Institute paid for the review, no author declared any conflict of interests. If ever there was a clear case of collusion with a view to distorting the truth, then this is it between the aluminum industry, the journal *JTEH*, and the publishers T&F. The main reason why I pursued the truth about this review is its shoddy nature and totally selected use of the published scientific literature. It essentially ignored all published science that implicated human exposure to aluminum in disease and especially those of the brain.

As I have already mentioned, this so-called review was designed as a smokescreen and a distraction from the real issues associated with human exposure to aluminum. The aluminum industry commissions and arranges publication of these sham papers about every decade or so, beginning with Sorensen et al. in 1974.[4] The fact that they are able to do so is testament to their power over the establishment and, in this case, the publishing industry specifically. When I see this review cited in manuscripts that I am reviewing, I point out its problems to authors. My efforts have not prevented the review from being cited several hundred times to date. Numbers of citations are usually interpreted as a mark of the quality of a scientific paper. This is what I meant earlier when I wrote about naive scientists researching aluminum. They believe they are citing a legitimate scientific paper.

In another example of how publishers, this time Elsevier, are heavily influenced by external forces, I recall how one day I came across, essentially out of the blue, a published Letter to the Editor about a paper I coauthored in the journal *Toxicology*. The notorious provaccine troll David Hawkes

---

4 John R. J. Sorenson, Irene R. Campbell, Lloyd B. Tepper, and Robert D. Lingg, "Aluminum in the Environment and Human Health," *Environmental Health Perspectives* 8 (1974): 3–95, https://ehp.niehs.nih.gov/doi/pdf/10.1289/ehp.7483.

JOURNAL OF
TOXICOLOGY AND
ENVIRONMENTAL HEALTH
Part B: Critical Reviews

Editor-in-Chief
SAM KACEW, Ph.D.
Department of Pharmacology
University of Ottawa
451 Smyth Road
Ottawa, Ont. K1H 8M5 Canada
Phone: (613) 562-5800 ext. 8357
Fax: (613) 562-5476
E-mail: skacew@uottawa.ca

Associate Editors:

KULBIR S. BAKSHI
Committee on Toxicology
Board on Environmental Studies and Toxicology
National Research Council/National Academy of Sciences
2101 Constitution Avenue, N.W.
Washington, DC 20418
(202) 334-2897
FAX: (202) 334-1393
Email: kbakshi@nas.edu

JANICE CHAMBERS
Center for Environmental Health Sciences
College of Veterinary Medicine
Mississippi State University
Box 9825
Mississippi State, MS 39762-9825
(662) 325-1255
FAX: (662) 325-1031
Email: chambers@novell.cvm.msstate.edu

SALLY D. PERREAULT
Reproductive Toxicology Division (MD-72)
National Health & Environmental Effects
    Research Laboratory
US EPA
Research Triangle Park, NC 27711
(919) 541-3826
FAX: (919) 541-4017
Email: darney.sally@epa.gov

RUDOLFS K. ZALUPS, PH.D.
Division of Basic Medical Sciences
Mercer University School of Medicine
1550 College Street
Macon, GA 31207 U.S.A.
(912) 301-2559
FAX: (912) 301-5489
Email: zalups.rk@gain.mercer.edu

February 14, 2007

Dr. Daniel Krewski
McLaughlin Centre for Population Health Risk Assessment
Institute of Population Health
University of Ottawa
1 Stewart Street , Room 318
Ottawa, Ontario
K1N 6N5

Re: MS # R-286

Title: Human health risk assessment...

Dear Dan:

I am happy to inform you that your manuscript has been accepted in its revised version and forwarded to our publishers Taylor & Francis for further handling. Your paper will appear in print in approximately 8 months. Taylor & Francis with the proofs of your paper approximately 6months prior to publication. Please note that the number of issues per year will increase in 2007 from 6 to 8 to speed-up the publication process,

Should any questions arise concerning galley proofs, the volume in which the article is to appear, etc., please contact Andrea McFadden(tel.215-625-8900   ext.213)   or   e-mail andrea.mcfadden@taylorandfrancis.com at Taylor and Francis.

Thank you for your interest in the Journal of Toxicology and Environmental Health.

Sincerely,

Sam Kacew, Ph.D.
Editor-in-Chief

Taylor & Francis
Taylor & Francis Group
www.taylorandfrancis.com

Figure 14. The editor of the *Journal of Toxicology and Environmental Health* accepting his own aluminium industry-funded manuscript for publication.

was one of the authors of the letter.[5] When I asked Editor-in-Chief Hans Marquardt why we were completely unaware of it and, as is usual practice, we had not been given the opportunity to reply to the letter prior to its publication, he answered in an email I have reproduced verbatim below:

> Dear Dr Exley,
>
> of course, you are absolutely right : I should have contacted you before publishing this letter. I have no explanation for this oversight. I sincerely apologize for this my mistake. I hope you can accept my apology.
>
> Best wishes YOURS Hans
> Professor Dr med Hans Marquardt

Subsequently, he offered us a retrospective right of reply that we accepted, and we submitted a rebuttal letter pointing out the true identities of the letter's authors and how they had purposely not declared their background affiliations as a conflict of interest. Our rebuttal letter, copied in full below, was, almost immediately and as promised, published by *Toxicology*. Once again, contrary to the usual rules, they did not show our letter to Hawkes and Benhamu or review it in any way prior to its publication:

Letter to the Editor

It is somewhat understating the case to say that we were surprised to learn of the publication by Toxicology of a Letter to the Editor (Hawkes & Benhamu, 2017) which addressed our recent publication in the same journal (Crepeaux et al., 2017). We had not been informed about this Letter and so we had not been offered any right of reply to the Letter. An apology for this 'oversight' has since been forthcoming from the Editor.

Letters to the Editor of a highly reputed journal such as Toxicology are considered as publications in their own right. In this respect we are not aware if the Letter by Hawkes and Benhamu was peer-reviewed? Our manuscript received rigorous peer review as would be expected and it might also be expected that any Letter questioning the scientific content of our published paper would be peer-reviewed and that this process would probably involve the original reviewers of our manuscript. If such a process had taken place it

---

5 Ghost Ship Media Facebook page, accessed October 1, 2020, https://www.facebook.com /ghostshipmedia.

is highly likely that the Letter by Hawkes and Benhamu would not have been published. Peer review would have established that the criticisms relating to our science were unfounded and only reflected the inexperience of the writers of this Letter in the field of aluminum adjuvants. We do not consider that we should now spend our time pointing out why the criticisms are either scientifically inept or simply ill-informed opinions. Again it is important to stress that our paper has already been thoroughly peer-reviewed by Toxicology unlike the Letter by Hawkes and Benhamu.

However, thorough peer-review of this Letter by Toxicology might have revealed the true motivation behind it. It would have revealed that the authors are both administrators and activists on behalf of a lobby group (Stop Australia's (anti) Vaccine Network, SAVN) and spend a considerable amount of time criticising in print (usually in non-peer-reviewed blogs such as The Conversation) anyone or any group that publishes excellent and peer-reviewed science criticising the safety record of human vaccines. Hawkes and Benhamu must have been delighted when the highly esteemed journal Toxicology published their Letter, their attempt to blur the evidence that the toxicokinetics of aluminum adjuvants are very poorly understood and deserve in depth evaluation.

In their Letter, Hawkes and Benhamu suggest that we have not been straightforward about our connections with the not-for-profit organisation, Children's Medical Safety Research Institute (CMSRI). We made it clear in the paper that the study was part-funded by the French Drug Agency ANSM, by CMSRI and by the University of British Columbia. Since none of us receive any form of 'financial compensation' (to use their phrase) from our roles on CMSRI's Scientific Advisory Board, we deemed that such was sufficient in respect of possible conflict of interests.

Readers of Toxicology may like to note that neither Hawkes nor Benhamu revealed their clear conflict of interests, namely their involvement with the SAVN lobby group. Actually Hawkes and Benhamu were purposely vague in respect of their affiliations in that Hawkes suggests, incorrectly, that he is currently a staff member at the University of Melbourne and neither of the affiliations given by Benhamu have even heard of her! The use of these reputable affiliations as a front was clearly an attempt to deceive the Editor in believing that the authors of the Letter were credible.

The co-authors of Crepeaux et al. are all scientists and we all seek the truth even if such may be unpalatable to some. We do the best science that we can with the funding that is available and we subject it to the most rigorous peer review as we did in the case of this paper. We welcome open and constructive criticism and we expect the journals that publish our research to treat it with the respect it deserves. Unfortunately through an apparent 'editorial oversight' such was not the case this time.

Crepeaux, G., Eidi, H., David, M.O., Baba-Amer, Y., Tzavara, E., Giros, B., Authier, F.J., Exley, C., Shaw, C.A., Cadusseau, J., Gherardi, R.K., 2017. Non-linear dose-response of aluminium hydroxide adjuvant particles: selective low dose neurotoxicity. Toxicology 375, 48–57.

Hawkes, D., Benhamu J., 2017. Questions about methodological and ethical quality of a vaccine adjuvant critical paper. Toxicology 389, 53–54.

Professor Christopher Exley (on behalf of all authors)
The Birchall Centre, Lennard-Jones Laboratories, Keele University,
Staffordshire, United Kingdom. c.exley@keele.ac.uk

Not long after the publication of our rebuttal letter, we received an email from someone called Mihail Grecea, a so-called publishing ethics expert at Elsevier. As you will see below, not only was Hawkes and Benhamu's letter about our research not peer-reviewed by *Toxicology*, but neither was our rebuttal. Elsevier had published our letter without reviewing its content until it was published. The email from Grecea informed us that our letter would now need to be withdrawn, as it included false information concerning Hawkes's affiliation. We had pointed out in our letter that Hawkes had used the University of Melbourne as his affiliation in his letter and not his actual full-time employment at the Victoria Cytology Service, a private company promoting and selling the HPV vaccine. Before making this assertion in our rebuttal letter, I had investigated Hawkes's claim to be a member of staff at the University of Melbourne. I searched for his name using the University's website search option and found no evidence of him. Allowing my curiosity to get the better of me, I then asked various contacts at the University of Melbourne, and specifically those in the department he cited in his affiliation, if Hawkes was currently a staff member. Curiously, I did not receive a single reply from anyone I emailed on the staff at the departments listed by Hawkes as his affiliations. Finally, an extensive search on the web revealed that Hawkes is not listed as a staff member of any department at the University of Melbourne. When all of this detailed information was sent to Mihail Grecea at Elsevier, they replied by sending us a link to the

University of Melbourne's "Find An Expert" website where Hawkes's affiliation with a division within the University, Pharmacology and Therapeutics, is listed as "honorary." This honorary affiliation is also not an active web link on this somewhat peripheral website. Under no circumstances, at the time of writing the letter to *Toxicology*, was Hawkes a current member of staff at the University of Melbourne. I think that most reading this information would conclude that our allusion to Hawkes being somewhat liberal with the truth about his connections to the University of Melbourne was correct. However, Elsevier did not see it this way and insisted that our letter be withdrawn. It should be noted at this point that Elsevier's "publishing ethics expert" Mihail Grecea found nothing untoward in any other aspect of this charade, including Hawkes's nondisclosure of his clear conflicts of interests and the barrage of editorial errors made by Hans Marquardt and Elsevier's publishing team. Only we, apparently, were in error.

While very unhappy with this decision, I suggested that the only fair outcome would be if both Hawkes's letter and our reply letter were withdrawn. I received the following reply from Kendall Wallace, then the coeditor, now editor-in-chief, of *Toxicology*.

> Prof. Exley,
>
> Let me introduce myself as co-editor with Prof. Marquardt for the Elsevier journal Toxicology. I corresponded with Prof. Marquardt Wednesday and we both agree with your latest email that Dr. Hawke's letter should be retracted as well. Prof. Marquardt is presently preoccupied with other matters and some of the Elsevier staff has left for the Holidays, so it may be that we won't be able to execute this retraction as quickly as we would hope. However, I assure you of our intentions and that both Hans and I will be working with Elsevier over the next few days to submit a letter of retraction as soon as possible.
>
> I hope this satisfies any concerns you may have. Thank you,

Within just a few days of my receipt of this email, with Hans Marquardt hurriedly retired by the journal and no longer replying to any emails, Kendall Wallace went back on his decision to retract the Hawkes letter and did so without providing us with any reason. Indeed, he never corresponded with me directly about this decision. He, the editor-in-chief of the renowned journal *Toxicology*, was clearly embarrassed by being forced by someone in Elsevier to change his previous position. To steal and paraphrase an appropriate quotation from the great English Bard, Shakespeare, "something was very rotten indeed in the state of Elsevier," and it remains so to this day.

Hawkes is a perennial spoiler, and one can only wonder as to his motivation. However, he does seem to be plying his trade to open-eared publishers and editors. Allow me to recall another very recent example of his stock-in-trade. Following a number of repeated invitations, I eventually agreed to be guest editor of a special issue, *Aluminum Adjuvants, Vaccines and Adverse Events*, for the publisher MDPI:

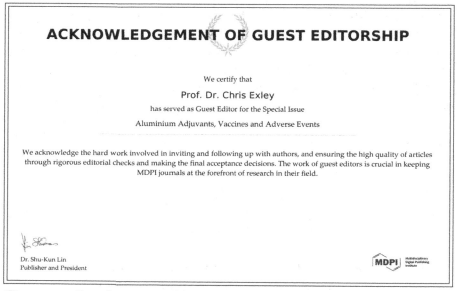

Figure 15. Certificate issued by the publisher MDPI for the special issue "Aluminum adjuvants, vaccines and adverse events."

We had previously published three papers with this publisher, and at this time I had assumed from the address of their headquarters that they were a Swiss-based company. Only later did I find out that MDPI is a Chinese company. Those who know me well are aware of my objections, based on human rights issues, to working with or supporting the Chinese regime (not individuals). After I accepted the offer to guest-edit a special issue, the publisher then produced a web page for the special issue with a description of the aims of the issue and all other relevant information about submission and deadlines and so forth. However, almost immediately, I smelled the rat that had previously pissed on my Elsevier *Toxicology* parade as editors at MDPI handling submissions to the special issue began, in their broken Chinese English, to insinuate that contributing authors were anti-vaccine. At first, I was perplexed as to where these insinuations had originated. However, as guest editor, I had access to the journal's peer review system, and I immediately came across the name of Hawkes as a reviewer chosen by the publisher. Here was the perpetrator of these lies. However, while I endeavored to inform the various handling editors that Hawkes was no more than an HPV vaccine salesman and an Internet troll, and therefore unsuitable as a reviewer of science, they chose to ignore my advice.

Faced with this uncomfortable situation, I decided to withdraw as guest editor and asked MDPI to remove my special issue from their advertising and website. Somewhat frustrated if not entirely surprised by this turn of events, I set about finding new homes for those few manuscripts that had already been submitted to the now-canceled special issue. Not long thereafter, another case of serendipity confirmed that which I had already supposed. An Achilles' heel of vaccine trolls, like Hawkes, is that they cannot help but celebrate their perceived victories with other similar trolls. Freedom of Information requests concerning another matter revealed Hawkes's celebrations with Dorit Reiss. The latter, a renowned vaccine troll, sent a reply email to Hawkes saying, "Congratulations!" The subject heading of the email Reiss is replying to is "Concerns about special issue Aluminum Adjuvants, Vaccines and Adverse Events," this being the subject heading of an email originally sent by Hawkes to the editor-in-chief, Paul Tchounwou, of the MDPI journal hosting the special issue. In this email, dated July 7, 2019, Hawkes helpfully points out to Tchounwou that I (Dr. Exley) am being manipulated by known antivaccine scientists to get their discredited research published in a creditable journal. One day later, the estimable Tchounwou passes on Hawkes's concerns to a managing editor at MDPI, Bonnie Wang, asking her to investigate his claims. Within a week, Wang is writing to Hawkes and Tchounwou, email dated July 15, to announce that she has taken action to remove the special issue from the journal. Ms. Wang is lying. I never received any correspondence from anyone at MDPI concerning removal of the special issue. I wrote to the editors dealing with the special issue on the July 11, 2019 to ask that the special issue be withdrawn. Why Ms. Wang, representing the publisher MDPI, chose to lie to Tchounwou and Hawkes about this is again open for debate but does not endear one to the publisher.

Hawkes responds to the email from Wang by sending himself an email in which he writes "Ka pow First time I have managed to have a special issue removed!" This email by Hawkes to "self" is the one received by Dorit Reiss and no doubt other vaccine troll associates. I wrote to Tchounwou and Wang, offering them an opportunity to defend their actions, but neither replied. Hawkes and his bcc'd cronies will no doubt be disappointed to learn that all papers destined for the special issue are now published in first class journals. His victory was very short-lived, but it is yet another example of how journals and publishers are being dictated to by external disruptive forces. In this case, the editor-in-chief, Tchounwou, was more than willing to have the wool pulled over his eyes by Hawkes, seemingly preferring his opinion to that of my own in this matter. I hope that my unanswered emails to him on this matter at the very least have caused him some personal embarrassment.

There are, unfortunately, many examples of openly corrupt journal editors supported by their publishers. Take for example the editor of *Academic Pediatrics*, Peter Szilagyi.

The manuscript that I have copied in full below was sent to the editor of the Elsevier journal *Academic Pediatrics* but was subsequently returned by the editor with the note that the journal does not publish "Letters" about papers published in the journal. When I asked the editor about other ways to address the scientific flaws in this paper, he did not reply. You can read about the editor of *Academic Pediatrics* and come to your own conclusions as to why such a fundamentally flawed paper was published with his full support.[6] I also sent the below manuscript to the lead author of the paper, Alan Woolf, but without any reply. Authors, friendly editors, and agenda-driven publishers collude at the expense of science all too often.

---

6   "Peter G. Szilagyi, MD, MPH," UCLA Health, accessed October 1, 2020, https://www.uclahealth .org/peter-szilagyi.

Letter to the Editor of Academic Pediatrics:
The Safety of Aluminum Adjuvants in Infants

In a recent paper by Woolf and colleagues[7], an attempt is made to connect the body burden of aluminum to aluminum exposure through vaccination and how these might impact upon early infant development. The laudable working hypothesis being to establish if exposure to aluminum through vaccination is affecting early infant development. The authors conclude that it is not. I find the research described in this paper at best unconvincing and at worst seriously flawed. The provenance of the major issues is probably a lack of experience and understanding by the paper's authors of aluminum in human health. For example, the authors used two indices of human exposure to aluminum, hair and whole blood, neither of which are widely accepted as reliable indicators of the body burden of aluminum[8]. Attempts were then made to relate these data with aluminum exposure through vaccines, the latter calculated erroneously as if all adjuvant aluminum administered in a vaccine dissolves into the whole body of an infant equilibrating, presumably, with whole blood and hair[9]. The authors also appear to assume that adjuvant aluminum will be the only significant source of aluminum to infants, somehow forgetting that infant formulas are heavily contaminated with aluminum[10]. Indeed breast milk may also be a significant source of aluminum to the infant[11].

The data obtained for hair aluminum can largely be discarded as, regardless of numerous published studies, hair aluminum remains to be demonstrated as a useful biological index of human exposure to aluminum. Whole blood, as opposed to serum, may, in the future following robust validation, prove to be useful in estimating the body burden of aluminum but not in this

7 MP Karwowski, C Stamoulis, LM Wenren, et al., "Blood and hair aluminum levels, vaccine history and early infant development: A cross sectional study," *Academic Pediatr* 18 (2018): 161–165.

8 C. Exley C, "Human exposure to aluminum," *Environ. Sci. Proc. Impacts* 15 (2013): 1807–1816.

9 JD Masson, G Crépeaux, F-J Authier, C Exley, and RK Gherardi, "Critical analysis of reference studies on the toxicokinetics of aluminum-based adjuvants," *J. Inorg. Biochem* 181 (2018): 87–95.

10 N Chuchu, B Patel, B Sebastian, and C Exley, "The aluminum content of infant formulas remains too high," *BMC Pediatrics* 13 (2013): 162.

11 D Fanni, R Ambu, C Gerosa, et al, "Aluminum exposure and toxicity in neonates: a practical guide to halt aluminum overload in the prenatal and perinatal periods," *World J. Pediatr* 10 (2014):101–107.

study due to significant issues in relation to its measurement. For example, no details are given as to how blood was collected. Researchers are often unaware that commercially available blood collection devices are heavily contaminated with aluminum leading to significantly higher measured values, as indeed are observed in this study. If, as is suggested in this paper, method blanks employing distilled water were used then, in the first instance, distilled water is not an appropriate blank for these preparations and secondly the method blank data obtained should be reported along with how they were used in any adjustments of final values. The authors report that they used a blood volume of (as little as) 0.1 mL which following digestion was diluted to a final volume of 5 mL. A dilution factor of 50 which when applied to their median blood aluminum content of 15.4 µg/L means that they were measuring 0.31 µg/L as their median value using an instrument which they suggest had a limit of detection of 0.1 µg/L. The measurement of aluminum in human tissues is fraught with problems and demands the highest levels of quality assurance[12]. Primary data should be adjusted appropriately with representative method blanks and while I cannot say that the data presented in this paper are erroneous much about their provenance and final values suggests that they might not be reliable. The authors also concede as much in their discussion.

One does wonder why the authors believed that whole blood (and hair) would be reliable indicators of infant exposure to aluminum through vaccination. The current consensus is that urinary excretion of aluminum, either 24h or creatinine-corrected spot values, is the best estimate of the body burden of aluminum[13]. Unfortunately, such data are not yet available for infants in the age group of this study. However, it must be debatable if aluminum exposure solely through vaccination would even be discernible using urinary excretion considering infants' additional exposure to aluminum through formulas and occasionally breast milk. In addition, the assumption that adjuvant aluminum is metabolised in the body in the same way as that entering the body in feed through the gut seems somewhat far-fetched. The fate of aluminum in the human body is very much governed by the original route of exposure[14]. Adjuvant aluminum is known to be harvested at vaccine injection sites by immune reactive cells many of which are very long lived and are capable

12 House, Esiri, Forster, Ince, and Exley, "Aluminium, iron and copper in human brain tissues donated to the medical research council's cognitive function and ageing study," *Metallomics.*
13 C Exley, "Human exposure to aluminium," *Environ. Sci. Proc. Impacts* 15 (2013): 1807–1816.
14 Exley, "The toxicity of aluminium in humans/La toxicité de l'aluminium chez l'homme," *Morphologie.*

of transporting aluminum throughout the body[15]. A recent publication on aluminum in brain tissue in autism demonstrated that the fate of such cells might be the brain[16].

The authors are not correct in their assertion that the safety of aluminum adjuvants in infants has been well established[17]. No such experiments on the safety of aluminum adjuvants have ever been carried out, nor is there currently any regulatory requirement for such. Paediatric vaccines that include an aluminum adjuvant are tolerated by the majority of recipients, though longer term effects or consequences have not been investigated, while some infants do experience serious adverse events which remain largely unexplained[18]. The authors' use of 'internet' citations (10-12 in the paper) in an attempt to belittle the potential dangers of aluminum adjuvants is unbecoming and should have been questioned during peer review. The authors are correct in their assertion that the safety of aluminum adjuvants in pediatric vaccines demands attention, unfortunately this study achieves very little in this respect.

Professor Christopher Exley PhD FRSB
The Birchall Centre, Lennard-Jones Laboratories, Keele University,
Staffordshire, United Kingdom. c.exley@keele.ac.uk

This flawed paper by Woolf and colleagues is repeatedly cited by those looking to support the safety of pediatric vaccines. By refusing to even peer-review a letter on the paper's failings, the editor, Szilagyi, and publisher, Elsevier, are colluding with the authors to protect its erroneous conclusions. This is why I am publishing my view of this paper in this book so that the alternative view is available for wider scrutiny.

15 M Mold, H Eriksson, P Siesjö, A Darabi, E Shardlow, and C Exley, "Unequivocal identification of intracellular aluminum adjuvant in a monocytic THP-1 cell line," *Scientific Reports* 4 (2014): 6287; Z Khan, C Combadière, FJ Authier, et al., "Slow CCL2-dependent translocation of biopersistent particles from muscle to brain," BMC Medicine 11 (2013): 99.

16 M Mold, D Umar, A King, C Exley, "Aluminum in brain tissue in autism," *J. Trace Elem. Med. Biol.* 46 (2018): 76–82.

17 JD Masson, G Crépeaux, F-J Authier, C Exley, and RK Gherardi, "Critical analysis of reference studies on the toxicokinetics of aluminum-based adjuvants," *J. Inorg. Biochem.*

18 JM Glanz, SR Newcomer, MF Daley, et al., "Cumulative and episodic vaccine aluminum exposure in a population-based cohort of young children," *Vaccine* 33 (2105): 6736–6744.

Closer to Home

I have had to deal with the consequences of politics in aluminum research for the majority of my academic career. Every paper published and every grant won has been a battle, and in some ways the resulting portfolio of science is the better for these battles. I have been fortunate in that, for the most part, I have had the full support of my university. Unfortunately, this unconditional support was abruptly removed about five years ago.

I have been a scientist at Keele University since June 1992. The great majority of my science has been carried out at Keele, and this body of research, recorded in over two hundred papers, has secured my reputation as Mr. Aluminum. I have enjoyed open support and encouragement from Keele for all but the last five years or so. Changes in appreciation of my research group efforts have been coincident with a new guard in senior management at Keele and, you may not be surprised to hear, funding from the Bill and Melinda Gates Foundation and the arrival on campus of an outlet of Well, the United Kingdom's largest independent pharmacist. The latter has involved a number of significant collaboration's with Keele's Department of Pharmacy, including joint staff appointments. There was also a time when Well was allowed to use Keele's intranet to sell vaccines to staff and students. I questioned this practice, allowing a commercial organization access to Keele's private messaging service, and though my question remained unanswered, it does appear to have had the desired effect of stopping this unwanted and divisive commercial practice. The first solid indication I had that Keele was no longer prepared to support my research openly was censorship by the faculty dean of a press release. The same Dean had, just days before, approved the original press release, and it had been posted on Keele's website. Just two days later, the content of the release had been changed without any prior consultation with me. Only a risible explanation for the about-face in the dean's approval was offered, and it then transpired that neither the original nor the censored press release had even been sent out externally. It was a press release that was not released to the press. Once again, a complaint directed toward the vice-chancellor at Keele was not even acknowledged. The censored press release is still available through the University's website.[19] I am reproducing the text that was removed from the concluding section of the release:

---

19 "How might aluminium adjuvants contribute towards vaccine-related adverse events?" August 15, 2016, https://www.keele.ac.uk/research/researchnews/2016/howmightaluminium adjuvantscontributetowardsvaccine-relatedadverseevents.php.

Professor Exley adds that there are no clinically-approved aluminum adjuvants only clinically approved vaccines which use aluminum adjuvants. This makes it imperative that all vaccine trials which use aluminum salts as adjuvants must not use the aluminum adjuvant as the control or placebo. This has been common practice for many years and has resulted in many vaccine-related adverse events due in part or in entirety to aluminum adjuvants being unaccounted for in vaccine safety trials.

Someone, almost certainly external to the University, took umbrage at the content of this paragraph and had sufficient sway with the University hierarchy for it to be removed from the press release without any discussion with me first. Take note that at this time the risible reason given by the dean for removing the text was that it was poor written English. This press release, which was not released to the press, is dated August 2016, and it is the last time that Keele University featured my group's research, internally or externally, in any format. In spite of our publishing a number of seminal studies on, for example, autism and Alzheimer's disease, our research has not been featured internally at Keele, never mind being released to the national and international press. The decision by Keele to actively ignore our research and to dissuade others from covering it is particularly damaging for the two young, first-class scientists working with me, Dr. Matthew Mold and Dr. Emma Shardlow. They are to be commended for continuing their groundbreaking work in the face of such lack of support from their University. By way of an example of Keele's extreme response to our work: when the *Journal of Alzheimer's Disease* produced a press release on our recent research on familial Alzheimer's disease,[20] including a strongly supportive comment from the editor-in-chief, Professor George Perry, Keele chose not to feature the work. When I questioned this decision, the pro-vice chancellor for Research at Keele called the research "unremarkable" and my personal comments on the subject area of aluminum and Alzheimer's disease "egregious."

On a number of occasions, this same individual has acted to impede, unsuccessfully, the progress of our research. In a meeting with him, I once asked him to his face to be transparent—indeed honest, in his actions, at least—in private with myself. If Keele was under pressure from significant external partners and investors to downplay the research coming from my

20 "Human Exposure to Aluminum Linked to Familial Alzheimer's Disease," January 20, 2020, https://www.j-alz.com/content/human-exposure-aluminum-linked-familial-alzheimer%E2%80%99s-disease.

group, then, I asked, simply tell me this. I could then at least understand this position even if I might not agree with it. However, he refused any such transparency, at least until very recently and not with me directly.

As many of you will be aware, donations play a very large part in funding our scientific research. They are the lifeblood of my group. Recently, I was very pleased to receive a donation from Robert F. Kennedy, Jr., the famous environmental campaigner and the nephew of past US president John F. Kennedy. I felt honored to receive such a donation, and I assumed that Keele would similarly covet recognition from such an esteemed family. I could not have been further from the mark. Once again, the pro-vice chancellor for Research, on behalf of Keele, was involved in rejecting the donation. The reasons for which were given as not wishing to jeopardize strong relationships with existing major funders and partners. Here for the first time, either in print or spoken, is the admission by senior management at Keele that external forces are dictating academic freedom at Keele. This is in many ways an astonishing admission, and whether the pro-vice chancellor realized what he was writing in the letter to Robert F. Kennedy, Jr., is uncertain.

Such an admission also raises significant issues of double standards. While Keele considers a modest donation from a prominent environmental campaigner as too controversial, they were more than happy to accept a donation of nine million pounds from the locally established online betting company Bet365 to build a management center. The new building is one of the first seen upon entering the Keele campus and is emblazoned with the name of Bet365's chief executive officer, Denise Coates. Keele's role in advertising the "good" in online betting smacks of general practitioners' in a bygone age promoting smoking cigarettes as "good for the nerves." The fact that neither Keele's hierarchy nor any of its major funders and partners objected to such a large donation from an industry beset with major problems of human addictive behavior is testimony to the nature of those currently dictating academic freedom at Keele. RFK Jr.'s views on the actions of Keele have been eloquently presented in a Children's Health Defense article.[21]

---

21 Robert F. Kennedy, Jr., "Is Pharma Censoring the Science at One Major University by Choking the Money Channel?" *Children's Health Defense*, April 29, 2020, https://childrenshealthdefense .org/news/is-pharma-censoring-the-science-at-one-major-university-by-choking-the-money -channel/.

I have spent over twenty-eight years building and establishing my laboratory at Keele, and for the most part the University has encouraged and supported me. I have attracted in excess of five million pounds of research funding, and we have used this to contribute world-class research published in over 200 papers. Keele is my University, and not having the support of the current senior management is not a reason to disown Keele. While the lack of senior management support for our research saddens me, I have experienced many different working environments over my tenure here at Keele, and the next new broom may well choose to support, encourage, and celebrate our research. The best way to ensure this happens is to continue to bring in research funding and use this to produce the very best research output. Politics is ephemeral and moves with whichever taste is blowing in the wind. Good science, though always evolving, is not prone to political and personal whims. It often does stand the test of time. I intend to do just that here in the Birchall Centre at Keele University.

Putting to one side the puerile activities of vaccine trolls such as Gorski and Hawkes, it is probably true to say that issues of prejudice and censorship thus far encountered have not been of a personal nature. Well, that was before I recently, in spring 2020, agreed to be interviewed by an organization called People Behind the Science.[22]

The cofounder of this organization, Marie McNeely, contacted me by email and convinced me to take part in an interview. I suppose that it was my immodesty that won the day, since McNeely assured me that the interview would be more about me, the scientist, than my research. The telephone interview went well. I was unusually candid and probably gave away a little more than I might have originally intended. In a follow-up email, McNeely expressed her pleasure with the interview and informed me that it would be broadcast through their podcast in a few weeks. Just a few days ago, I received an email from someone called Michael Green, another cofounder of the organization. He informed me that they would not be broadcasting the interview. He offered no explanation. I sent an email to McNeely, and while she replied, no explanation was forthcoming.

Since the interview contained personal information about myself and would not now be used as originally intended, I asked for the tape of the interview to be returned to me. Personally, I have had no replies to date from either Green or McNeely. However, when my US-based lawyer approached

---

22 *People Behind the Science* home page, accessed October 1, 2020, http://www.peoplebehind thescience.com/.

them, they did reply, and an offer was made to return a version of the taped interview.[23] It was not what we had expected!

Since this organization has editorial control and could edit the tape of the conversation, as they deemed appropriate, I have to interpret their actions as censorship of me. They knew all about my research when they invited me for the interview, and yet something happened post-interview to change their minds. Something or someone intervened, perhaps one of the platforms for their podcast. Their silence on this matter and refusal to return the complete tape of the interview has sinister connotations. Do feel free to ask them why they censored Professor Christopher Exley PhD FRSB.

---

23 "The Censorship of Professor C Exley PhD FRSB," accessed October 1, 2020, https://www.youtube.com/watch?v=XUTJWwy-KiI&t=1076s.

CHAPTER 20

Imagine You Are an Aluminum Atom

Stealing a few words from the great Neil Young as he joined The Band for "The Last Waltz," I would like to say that it has been one of the pleasures of my life to share the scientific stage with so many wonderful people. In choosing science over business, as I eventually did about thirty-five years ago, I had accepted that the riches in my life would need to be found away from financial interests. This aspiration, I am pleased to report, turned out to be true many times over, and one of those riches is the propensity to travel and meet fascinating people, some scientists and some becoming lifelong friends. The title of this chapter and the book comes from one such meeting. Through the Keele Meetings on Aluminum,[1] I had become acquainted with an exceptional group of computational chemists led by Jesus Ugalde (affectionately known by me as El Presidente), who is based in San Sebastian, Spain. They invited me to give a talk at a theoretical biophysics symposium in Sweden, and, unbeknown to me at the time, the opening line of my talk, "Imagine you are an aluminum atom," caused some mirth among the mainly theoretical computational chemists in the audience. Over a rare beer—we were in "outer-Sweden" where beer is both rare and expensive—an outstanding young chemist, Xabier Lopez, explained to me the novelty of such an expression, at least in that particular company. Dr. Lopez is now Professor Lopez and, in my opinion, the leading computational aluminum chemist in the world and, I am proud to say, a great friend. I have a specific

1 Bioinorganic Chemistry of Aluminium & Silicon, Keele Meetings, accessed October 1, 2020, https://www.keele.ac.uk/aluminium/keelemeetings/.

memory of this event and, indeed, my statement because it is an accurate reflection of my problem-solving abilities. I have always approached questions in science as thought experiments. If I cannot picture the science in my mind, then I cannot begin to understand a problem and how it can be solved. If I can share my imaginative approach with myriad scientists in multiple, sometimes wonderful, locations, then all the better. If you decide to read this book, then you will know who you are, how you have impacted my life and my science. Many of you are valued collaborators and coauthors. Thank you.

Another moment that I would like to share with you also happened at one of the Keele Meetings on Aluminum.[2] I remember some of this occasion very well. I can see the lecture room in my mind's eye and my old friend Paolo Prolo giving a presentation on the economic cost of Alzheimer's disease. I think it was the Seventh Keele Meeting, 2007, which was the first time the meeting was held in Uxmal, Mexico. We returned to this magical venue in March 2019 for the Thirteenth Keele Meeting on Aluminum. Toward the end of Paolo's talk, or perhaps even in the discussion period that followed, Paolo let it slip for the first time, at least to my knowledge, that I was known among the aluminum family as Mr. Aluminum.

At first this took me aback, as I really had not heard this term used previously by anyone. Quickly it transpired that it was a term used as a mark of respect and also affectionately, and I was quick to embrace its meaning. Mr. Aluminum has meant a lot to me over subsequent years, and I have endeavored to live up to such a moniker. If at least some of the aluminum family recognize my efforts through such an accolade, then I am proud to be Mr. Aluminum.

Being Mr. Aluminum has been my full-time employment since 1984, when the aluminum seed was somehow planted in my brain. The nourishment of this seed, that which has allowed it to grow and become Mr. Aluminum, has depended upon myriad individuals, too many to thank individually here. It has also depended upon financial support without which Mr. Aluminum would have, as they say, withered on the vine. During the past ten years, financial support from one individual in particular has meant the difference between the continuation of groundbreaking research, as documented in this book, and no book. This person has not only funded our research, but she has also "imagined that she was an aluminum atom." She has embraced the subject and the science, and in doing so I am confident

---

2 Ibid.

that she feels that her dollars have been well spent. She is, of course, Mrs. Claire Dwoskin, the founder of the Children's Medical Safety Research Institute (CMSRI) in Washington, DC. With CMSRI funding acting as the foundations, we have continued to build our research home with many varied income, including especially wonderful donations from private individuals. These donations are the lifeblood of what we are doing now and I hope, if they continue, what we can do in the future. Thank you to all.

Finally, thank you for reading this heartfelt book. I have enjoyed sharing my aluminum journey with you, and as with all too-long journeys, your eyelids are probably feeling heavy and a light is about to be extinguished. Before you go, may I share with you a recent recurring dream of mine? I am in the grand lecture hall at the Royal Society, Carlton House Terrace, London[3] and looking down over a packed audience that is listening attentively to an excited speaker. There is no better place and no more conducive environment in which to report and receive the latest science. It is the home of British science and, arguably, world science. There is no greater accolade for a British scientist than to be invited to the Fellowship of the Royal Society and to have those letters, FRS, after your name. But I digress, let's go back to my dream. The gathering of scientists, and clearly some press, seemingly below me, is being made to wait for an all-important slide. Well, not a slide per se but simply a change in the content of the large white display board. A new infographic appears and an almost shocked, paralyzed even, silence ensues. The chair of the meeting, no less than the president of the Royal Society, sitting just to one side at the front of the hall, rises to her feet (the first female president, I think to myself) and begins to clap slowly and resolutely. Her colleagues on the front bench soon join her, and it is no more than seconds before everyone in the hall is on their feet and applauding enthusiastically. The scientist making the presentation makes an extended and somewhat dramatic bow. This seems to excite the audience further, and the clapping gets louder and the press have their pictures, destined this time for the front page. The information on the giant white screen drawing the plaudits is straightforward and unequivocal:

The number of individuals in the treatment group (10,000 across 10 centres around Europe), all previously diagnosed with mild cognitive impairment, who went on to develop Alzheimer's disease after 10 years was zero.

---

3 Royal Society home page, accessed October 1, 2020, https://royalsociety.org/.

It had taken almost one hundred and fifty years from the first diagnosis for science to conquer the scourge of Alzheimer's disease. The treatment? Nothing is actually said in my dream. However, from my lofty eyrie turning to my right, I catch the eye of someone I know, pipe in hand, a glint in his eyes, and a broad smile across his face.[4] Before I can catch myself saying to him, "Well Derek, we were right," I wake up with those words on my lips.

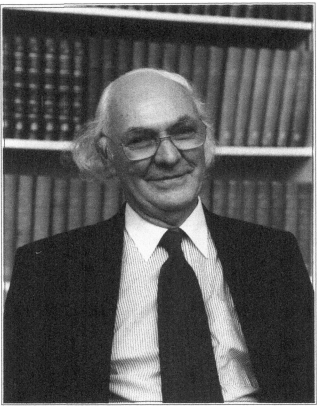

Figure 16. My "father-in-science," mentor, and great friend: the late JD Birchall OBE FRS.

4 Anthony Kelly and A. J. Howard, "James Derek Birchall, O. B. E. 7 October 1930–7 December 1995," *Biographical Memoirs of Fellows of the Royal Society* 43 (1997) https://royalsocietypublishing .org/doi/10.1098/rsbm.1997.0006.

ACKNOWLEDGMENTS

Thank you to the Aluminum Family. Your decades of tireless, under-funded, and often unappreciated research gave me the opportunity to write this book. My story is your story.